T0323144

EVERYTHING YOU NEED TO KNOW ABOUT THE PILL

GALLIMARD

EVERYTHING YOU NEED TO KNOW ABOUT THE PILL (BUT WERE TOO AFRAID TO ASK)

KATE MUIR

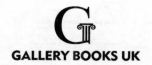

GALLERY BOOKS UK

First published in Great Britain by Gallery Books, an imprint of
Simon & Schuster UK Ltd, 2024

1 3 5 7 9 10 8 6 4 2

Simon & Schuster UK Ltd
1st Floor
222 Gray's Inn Road
London WC1X 8HB

Simon & Schuster: Celebrating 100 Years of Publishing in 2024

www.simonandschuster.co.uk
www.simonandschuster.com.au
www.simonandschuster.co.in

Simon & Schuster Australia, Sydney
Simon & Schuster India, New Delhi

Disclaimer:
This book is an investigation of hormonal contraception,
but it is not medical advice. Always consult your doctor.

A CIP catalogue record for this book is available from the British Library

Hardback ISBN: 978-1-3985-2951-9
eBook ISBN: 978-1-3985-2952-6

Typeset in Perpetua by M Rules
Printed and Bound in the UK using 100% Renewable Electricity at CPI
Group (UK) Ltd

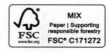

*In memory of the pioneering Dr Katharina Dalton
(1916–2004), who first identified and treated
premenstrual syndrome (PMS)*

CONTENTS

'Every woman has a militant responsibility to involve herself actively with her own health. We owe ourselves the protection of all the information we can acquire . . . '

Audre Lorde

CHAPTER ONE

PILL ROULETTE

The contraceptive pill needs no introduction. It is the most intimate of companions, lurking in handbags among lipsticked tissues; offering free love on bedside tables; hiding its shame in sock drawers. The pill's man-made synthetic hormones have coursed invisibly through women's veins and brains for over half a century, freeing us from reproduction and encouraging revolution. Those tiny pills were the ball bearings that rolled in the feminist movement, allowed female fighter pilots to skip periods in war zones, and the rest of us to have sex any time, any place, with anyone. For the first time, thanks to the pill, women made exponential leaps forward in work, educational and orgasmic equality. The late period was a thing of the past.

We love the pill – and we hate it. The majority of women – and some trans men and non-binary people – are happy on hormonal contraception. It keeps us free of offspring, makes life more convenient, and saves on truckloads of tampons. Some pills help eliminate the hormonal dips of premenstrual syndrome (PMS) and sometimes the more debilitating premenstrual dysphoric disorder (PMDD). You'll read about the positives in official contraception guides, less so the negatives, of which there is very little investigation – until now.

So, while the pill needs no introduction, we need far more insight into our relationship with it. We pop these mini hormone-bombs out of their foil packs into our bodies for ten, twenty or even thirty years, without knowing a smidgen of the science behind them. I speak for myself here; I had no idea until I started researching this book what the synthetic hormones in the contraceptive pill, patch, coil, ring, injection or implant could do to our moods, our sex drive, our vaginal microbiome, our brain structure, our future health, our instinctive attraction and even our sense of smell. Such potency is fascinating and frightening in equal measure. Women (and other people with ovaries) need to be empowered with this knowledge. They need a toolkit to understand which contraception might work best for them, what effects it could have, and what might be coming in the future. I hope *Everything You Need to Know About the Pill* will be that useful toolkit, as well as a manual for revolution.

THE INSIDIOUS EFFECT ON MENTAL HEALTH

As I listened to story after story when researching this book, what struck me most shockingly and bleakly was the effect of hormonal contraception on our mental health. While the pill vanquishes painful periods and premenstrual syndrome for millions of women, for millions of others it can bring unexplained stress, anxiety and depression, which is often met with gaslighting from everyone, including those in the medical profession. Like frogs dropped into warming water, unaware of their impending doom at boiling point, women who take the pill blame themselves and their circumstances for their ever-lowering mood. 'The pill picked at me a little bit every day. I lost something,' said Kirsty Keating, one of my interviewees. We'll hear more from Kirsty in Chapter 3, but quite simply she bounced on to the pill aged fourteen to help with her acne, and only discovered when she came off it in her thirties that it had been slowly turning her into a completely different person: depressed and introverted.

Who takes these momentous decisions to replace their natural hormones with synthetic ones for decades? Schoolgirls, mostly. And maybe their mums. In a recent UK survey, 64 per cent of women said they first went on the pill as teenagers, and 29 per cent were unable to even name the brand of pill they were on.[1] Let's be honest: if you'd asked me a few years ago what was in the bog-standard combined pill, I might have guessed estrogen and progesterone. Wrong. The answer is the synthetic estrogen, ethinylestradiol, and one of dozens of different synthetic progestins, each of which might have a more masculinising or feminising effect on your body and mind. There are only progestins in the 'mini-pill' or POP (progestin only pill). Ethinylestradiol and progestins are man-made versions of estrogen and progesterone, and rather like ultra-processed foods, they have some peculiar molecular additions, which sometimes have unnatural effects. I learned that the hard way.

Back in 2020, I considered myself well informed about hormones, given I was writing a book about the hormonal hell of the menopause and the positive effects of natural body-identical hormone replacement therapy (HRT). At that time, my daughter Molly's mood deteriorated into depression. She was twenty, and I put it down to the misery of lockdown, being forced home from the University of Edinburgh and the loneliness of the long-distance Zoomer. She had struggled with depression before, but this was next level. 'I felt like I couldn't speak. I thought that if I walked into another room, I'd infect people with my sadness,' Molly said afterwards. She attempted to get help. 'I tried the university counsellor first, but they could only offer a half-hour phone call because there was such an influx of people needing counselling.' I found an art therapist who was doing mainstream therapy online while we were all locked down, and she and Molly got on well.

Amid such extreme circumstances, we never thought to question the impact Molly's pill might be having. I still feel guilty that I was so cavalier about Molly going on hormonal contraception in the first place, but I didn't see any alternative. She was fifteen years old and had periods so heavy and painful they left her faint at school, or in bed with a hot water bottle. We went to see the practice nurse at our local surgery to ask for help, and she immediately suggested the combined contraceptive pill and mefenamic acid, a tablet which blocks inflammation and reduces pain during a period.

Molly remembered how she felt back then: 'If I started my period when I was at a friend's house, she'd offer me a tampon and it would be this tiny thing, and I knew either I'd have to go through half a box or I'd have to go home. I felt really embarrassed about it, so I'd often use tissue instead.' This kind of shame about large tampons was hilariously depicted in an episode of *Fleabag*, when writer and star Phoebe Waller-Bridge spots a man she'd previously slept with while shopping for a box of super-sized tampons.[2] Fleabag panics and scrabbles to swap the super-sized tampons for the regular ones. 'What're you getting?' the man asks her. 'Oh, just these for my tiny bleeding vagina!' she trills. 'Hot,' he replies. 'Hope it's a low flow,' he adds. 'Oh, it never is, it never is,' she answers.

Molly changed her brand of pill at university, and ended up on the cheapest NHS choice, Rigevidon (ethinylestradiol and the progestin levonorgestrel). Her low mood started to get worse, and then her prescription ran out. 'I thought because of all the Covid restrictions I wouldn't be able to get more, so I just stopped taking them. I do also chalk it up to laziness – I have the memory of a goldfish, so I'd always forget to take them, miss a day, or I'd be at my boyfriend's house and have missed the window. I took the morning-after pill three or four times that year.' But within a few weeks of stopping taking the combined pill, the darkness slowly lifted. Molly seemed full of energy and significantly happier. It took us a while to clock this, but nothing else had altered in her life.

It was only after I directly saw the effect of hormonal contraception on Molly's mental health that I remembered

I'd been on a pill with exactly the same ingredients as Rigevidon: Microgynon — a green foil packet, wee beige pills — when I was a student at the University of Glasgow. I'd felt a bit flat and somewhat spotty for four years, but it was tolerable, given my extra-curricular sexual activity. I only realised that the pill had also lowered my libido after I came off it and discovered the glories of the estrogenic ovulation peak, creatively and sexually. But how could I not have joined the dots between my 'meh' experience and Molly's more serious depression on a similar brand? I suppose because I had no idea until that moment how much the pill affected our brains as well as our ovaries.

Eventually, Molly swapped to the Kyleena hormonal coil, which releases that same progestin, levonorgestrel, directly into the womb, but in much smaller amounts, and it had no negative effect on her mood. In mysterious sync, her four flatmates also changed to the coil. 'Once one person said how much easier it was — that it's painful on the day of insertion, but then you get three to five years of not having to bother with it any more — we all jumped on the coil train. Pre-insertion, we all took copious amounts of paracetamol to fend off the worst of the pain. I have friends who are vehemently opposed to having any hormones in their system, so they have the copper coil, but that was never an option for me because of my heavy periods. If there was a no-hormone option that gave me less-heavy periods, I'd take it in a heartbeat. I still get excruciating cramps, but they happen less often.'

A PILL REVOLUTION BEGINS

This experience went from the personal to the political at home during the second Covid lockdown. As Molly and I started researching the pill and mental health, we were astonished by the lack of official acknowledgement of the problem, shrugged off as 'mood swings' in the medical literature. I'd previously made two radical menopause documentaries that also explored mental health, and I began thinking about pitching a contraception documentary to Channel 4, which eventually became *Davina McCall's Pill Revolution* in 2023. For the documentary, we commissioned a contraception survey of more than 4,000 diverse women (and some non-binary people) aged sixteen to forty-nine around the UK.[3] While most were happy with the contraception they were now on, a hefty 77 per cent of pill-users said they had experienced side effects, and a third said those were severe enough to stop them taking it. Indeed, 57 per cent said they were concerned about the effect of hormonal contraception on their mental health. For 36 per cent, the worst side effects were low mood, anxiety or depression, for 37 per cent it was weight gain. Finally, 21 per cent reported lowered sex drive. I think we can fairly say that 'side effects' are in fact massively mainstream, and of course some of us are more hormone-sensitive than others.

There are over 150 million people on the pill worldwide,[4] but prescriptions are falling year on year in the UK, America and Europe, as women turn to other forms of contraception or just leave it to chance. NHS data showed community pharmacies dispensed 7.2 million items of progestin-only and combined pills in 2022–2023, a significant decrease from the 8.5 million in 2014–2015. Abortions are rocketing. (My own view is that there's nothing wrong with an abortion; indeed, I discuss my own later on, but there are decidedly better methods of contraception.) The abortion rate in the UK is at the highest it has ever been since legalisation in 1967.[5] In America, despite new draconian restrictions introduced in some states after the overturning of Roe v. Wade, abortions are still on the rise as women cross state lines or buy pills by post.[6] With so much contraceptive choice, why are we not choosing contraception?

THE TECTONIC SHIFTS OF THE 'PILLQUAKE'

There are three tectonic shifts happening at once to create this earthquake in contraception, this 'pillquake'. The first is that women are realising they have been gaslighted by doctors for decades about the serious side effects of the hormonal pill, implant, coil, ring, injection and patch, and are generally told to keep calm and carry on. The second is the embracing of 'green sex', fertility and menstrual cycle apps that promise accuracy. The third is the growth of the morning-after pill and the at-home abortion pill.

This social change is happening at hyper-speed. Molly also showed me her feed on hormonal contraception on TikTok, which was as gripping as it was mind-blowingly inaccurate. Since then, the posts trashing hormonal birth control and plugging natural cycles have grown to millions of hits. Medical professionals are flailing, finding it hard to keep up as anger and frustration about being gaslighted about symptoms is amplified on TikTok and other social media. There, fears of synthetic hormones are fuelled, along with breathless endorsements by influencers of new 'green' contraceptive methods, like the Natural Cycles App.

For the Millennial and Gen Z generations, TikTok and Instagram are a consultation room without the white coats and with better music, and certain influencers are trusted sources. If you can research the ten best retinol-based face serums online, why not the best contraceptives? Social media is a place where science is turned into slogans, but it's also a place to question the status quo, rightly or wrongly. Either way, the algorithm has taken over and will change contraceptive behaviour for ever – as sure as eggs is eggs, as my mother used to say.

'Birth control is this generation's cigarettes,' says a woman on TikTok.[7] 'It's a class-one carcinogen,' continues the feed. 'When women start taking the pill, they get massively depressed,' says another. 'It was 99.9 per cent effective in ruining my life.' These are just some of the millions of comments about the pill online. Then there's the meme of girls opening pill packets and unfurling the huge side effects warning leaflet, snuggling down under it like a blanket. Those who have come off hormonal contraception and turned to fertility awareness apps give the impression of a world of joy and rainbows – and no accidents.

There's no real attempt to take down these TikTok posts

by the powers that be, despite 'Community Guidelines' that say otherwise, according to the NewsGuard Misinformation Monitor. They found in test searches that a fifth of posts contained misinformation[8] and that TikTok was much less accurate as a search engine than Google (duh). Jennifer Takhar of the ISG International School of Business in Paris recently published a paper with Anna Schneider-Kamp of the University of Southern Denmark on the reasons behind the increasing rejection of the pill in Western Europe.[9] Takhar told me: 'Our research shows that peers on social media are influencing young women's choices, and reshaping how they perceive risks and side effects. At the same time, social media is delegitimising the authority of health professionals.' Their team interviewed women in Denmark and Germany about their growing concerns voiced on social media, and the trend towards fertility awareness methods and 'green sex'. While the American hashtag is often #quittingbirthcontrol, the Germans have coined a great portmanteau word: #Pillenmüdigkeit, meaning pill fatigue.

The TikTokers and Instagrammers are on to something though: it is true that women's complaints have been downplayed by the medical establishment and our culture right from the beginning. In Chapter 12, we'll see how dangerously high doses of the pill were first tested by American doctors on 265 Puerto Rican women in 1956. Three died of 'unknown causes', possibly from strokes or clots caused by the overdose of synthetic progestins in that pill. Others who complained of dizziness, headaches and stomach pain were also quietly written out of the glowing report, which went to the US Food and Drug Administration to be rubber-stamped before the contraceptive pill was unleashed on the world. After all, the drug was a miracle; it was proven to prevent pregnancy in women and saved men from the minor discomfort of putting on a condom. Why shouldn't women suffer a few minor discomforts too for this freedom?

How long can we pretend that everything is perfect to a new generation who will source their information elsewhere and demand better? Here's the brisk entry on the NHS website[10] for any problems with the combined pill: 'Minor side effects include mood swings, nausea, breast tenderness and headaches – these usually settle down in a few months. There is no evidence that the pill will make you gain weight. There's a very low risk of serious side effects, such as blood clots and cervical cancer.' Super. But that's not what I've found in the next thirteen chapters. It's time to listen and to tell women's truth.

DON'T MENTION THE SIDE EFFECTS . . .

Again and again, I've seen gaslighting and downplaying of the pill's side effects, such as depression, weight gain, dry vaginas, sore breasts, wildly unpredictable bleeding and lowered libido, and even more serious dangers like an increased risk of blood clots, strokes and breast cancer. No wonder women are screaming out online and in conversation with each other. The reporting of scientific studies on contraception and synthetic hormones can be surprisingly biased, just as I discovered about hormone replacement therapy when I wrote my menopause book. Received wisdom is not necessarily very wise. Always read the bottom line, not just the headline on research papers. I've got the medical textbooks on contraception on my desk, I've read the NHS advice, the incisive and careful analysis of methods of contraception on the Faculty of Sexual and Reproductive Healthcare website, and none of it truly reflects the huge outpouring of frustration and suffering that often lasts for years because women and their doctors fail to connect their problems to the pill. It's not fair that harried NHS GPs or pharmacists have under ten minutes, sometimes on the phone or online, to help women take this momentous health decision.

Most of the testimonies in this book are of women struggling with hormonal contraception, and I realise there's bias in that. Obviously, the pill can be a miracle in helping some women with PCOS, endometriosis symptoms, acne or heavy periods that bring them to their knees, and the coil can help with bleeding from fibroids and even stop periods altogether. There are many lesbians and trans and non-binary people – more about that in Chapter 10 – who use the pill for other reasons than contraception. In sport, banishing periods is often essential for competition, and female footballers who find their anterior cruciate ligament tends to ping at the elastic estrogenic peak of their ovulation can apparently calm levels down with the pill.[11] But when, for balance, I asked women to send me their success stories on the pill, the stories were all much the same and a bit dull: it was convenient, life was normal and they'd been happily on it for years. As Leo Tolstoy says famously in the opening to his novel *Anna Karenina*: 'All happy families are alike; each unhappy family is unhappy in its own way.' It's much the same with the pill.

There is a utilitarian philosophy behind this silence on side effects, which is that the medical authorities don't want to scare the happy majority of women away from birth control, and I understand that. However, there's rarely an acknowledgement of the chaos, just a reassuring 'if side effects continue longer than three months, you may wish to change to another pill'. Then patients will often find themselves playing pill roulette, trying progestin-only pills, combined pills, and one brand after another to see if things improve, with no trusted information on the varying effects of each pill. Three months is a long time to be miserable, and a recent UK poll[12] showed 80 per cent of women had swapped brands at least once, and 16 per cent three times or more.

There are over forty brands of pill available, and there's no *Which?* users' guide available. Some pills have testosterone-like progestins in them, so they are more androgenic, and perhaps more likely to cause, say, a dry vagina, acne or low mood. Some other combined pills have more ethinylestradiol and more estrogenic progestins in them, which may cause breast tenderness and fluid retention among other side effects. I'll explain more about this in Chapter 2. But how do you know what to switch to?

It turns out that GPs in the UK can access an online 'Pill Ladder' guide,[13] which features columns showing the various pill brands and statements like: 'For LESS oestrogenic activity then move across ladders to the LEFT. For

LESS progestogenic activity then move across ladders to the RIGHT.' But I think many of us feel we've fallen off the ladder, and most of us had no idea it was there. 'Pill counselling is really bad, really poorly managed,' said Dr Annabel Sowemimo, who works as a sexual and reproductive health registrar in Leicester. 'The majority are just shoved on a tablet. The consultation isn't adequate. People don't understand what's in the pill, and that there are many different versions.'

I was also surprised to discover talking to doctors that sometimes two different brands of pill, which have the exactly same quantities of synthetic hormones, can affect women differently because of the composition with other additives. For instance, these are the additives in the cheapest 'first choice' Rigevidon combined pill: colloidal anhydrous silica, magnesium stearate, talc, maize starch, lactose monohydrate, sucrose, calcium carbonate, titanium dioxide (E171), copovidone, macrogol 6000, povidone carmellose sodium. Whereas the similar Microgynon also contains yellow ferric oxide pigment (E172) and povidone 90. Lactose may be worth checking for in pills if you're intolerant, but the quantities are microscopic. Still, it's worth knowing exactly what's in the packet.

WHAT ARE WOMEN'S REAL-LIFE EXPERIENCES OF THE PILL?

Alice Pelton is the founder of The Lowdown,[14] which is basically Tripadvisor for contraception, with more than 6,000 reviews with star ratings from women of different brands of contraception, plus up-to-date medical advice from doctors. Alice's own experience of endometriosis and trying seven different forms of contraception – including the combined pill, the progestin pill and the hormonal coil – radicalised her: 'I thought, this is not okay. Why are women expected to deal with these side effects and not be given much help on how to manage them and what methods to choose?' She was astounded that this life-changing decision is made by most women and their doctors in a few minutes (or just over-the-counter with a speedy consultation with a pharmacist), and she wanted to think of women as consumers with choices.

As menstrual cycle and contraceptive information apps like Clue and Flo grew worldwide, gaining millions of users, Alice set up The Lowdown website in London in 2019 and it is now expanding to America. 'This is like choosing a mortgage, and we need to give women the time, the data and the experience to really make the right decision for them.' Women can have a contraception consultation with an NHS-trained doctor through The Lowdown and buy the particular contraceptives they want. Having a trustworthy space to vent about side effects has also cheered a lot of women up, and the reviews veer slightly to the negative – the happy pill poppers are elsewhere. 'This is about honesty and shared experience, and accepting a woman feels like that it's a clusterfuck of problems. It makes them feel heard. This is women saying 'Did you feel that too? Yeah, I did,"' said Alice.

In a sign of the changing times, the fertility awareness method is the most popular method of contraception on the website, followed by the hormonal and copper coil, and Eloine is the top-rated brand of pill. The mental health aspect of hormonal contraception also struck Alice as the missing link for so many pill-users, particularly when it is dismissed. The expert review of studies at the Faculty of Sexual and Reproductive Healthcare says: 'Young people may be advised that hormonal contraception may be associated with mood changes but there is no evidence that hormonal contraceptives cause depression.'[15] 'Mood changes' doesn't quite cover how crap women actually feel. 'How is the jury out on low mood on the pill?' said Alice. 'You can walk into a café and ask five women and two will tell you they've had low mood on the pill.'

Of course, you can come across a fantastic healthcare professional who will acknowledge all this, have alternative suggestions, and will encourage you to keep notes of any changes and come back for another consultation if things are going wrong. If your family doctor is not an expert, it is often worth going to a local sexual health clinic or a charity like Brook or MSI Reproductive Choices in the UK, or Planned Parenthood in the US, who advise women on contraception day in and day out and have expertise on complicated cases.

We filmed sexual and reproductive health nurse consultant Simphiwe Sesane for the documentary at the MSI Reproductive Choices clinic in London, and she gave us a full and graphic tour of every contraceptive method, including the non-hormonal copper coil, and the new, smaller hormonal coils, which often work better for women who have not had children. I met Sesane through my menopause work, as she campaigns for equality on her Instagram @BlackNurses_Midwives_UK and makes entertaining contraception and sexual health videos. While Sesane works for a charity, many of her expert colleagues in other clinics are affected by cuts; the public health grant to local councils used to fund sexual health services in England and Wales was slashed by over £1billion – 24 per cent – over six years up until 2021.[16] Freedom of Information requests revealed contraceptive coil-fitting waiting lists of months in the UK, and some up to a year in parts of Devon and Northern Ireland.[17]

Despite the fact every £1 spent on contraception services saves public services in the UK £9 in the long run over ten years, clinics are being closed and run down.[18] But at least contraception is free here. The situation is much worse in America, where 11 per cent of women have no health insurance at all,[19] and others have to pay extra on top of insurance every time they go to the doctor. The cost of getting a hormonal coil fitted can be over $1,000, but the non-profit company Medicines360 has pioneered a cheaper hormonal coil, costing about $75, and works with charity clinics to make sure no one is more than $100 out of pocket if they are uninsured. But it's not surprising that so many struggle on with the cheaper pill.

In terms of coil fittings, which are infamously uncomfortable as you will see in Chapter 6, it's often better to go to a big clinic where experienced professionals like Sesane fit them swiftly every day. She is also working with the Reproductive Justice Initiative to get the combined contraceptive patch made transparent. Presently it is an unappetising pinkish-beige. 'Salmon!' said Sesane, slapping one on her brown skin. 'Not very inclusive, is it?' A petition went to the Evra patch manufacturers Gedeon Richter in 2023, but at time of writing there was no news of any colour change.

DECOLONISING CONTRACEPTION

The Reproductive Justice Initiative (originally Decolonising Contraception) was set up in 2018 by Dr Sowemimo, who I mentioned earlier, with other doctors, sex educators and campaigners. During her medical training, Dr Sowemimo began to see the extent to which the Black community was racially marginalised by the medical profession in many areas, including contraception, and she wrote the book *Divided: Racism, Medicine and Why We Need to Decolonise Healthcare*. 'We're addressing the additional barriers some groups face in accessing health services, and questioning the idea that some groups have more reproductive rights than others.'

In seven years of training, she has only met one other Black registrar working in sexual and reproductive health. 'Many of my colleagues have no idea this is a profound issue at all, no understanding historically of a racial dynamic that many still feel exists now.' She referred to the history of contraceptive eugenics and acts of cruelty perpetuated in the name of medical experiments on Black people in America and here, including sterilisation. 'Because of this legacy of Black people being treated badly by the medical profession, there is a lack of trust.' And although things are changing, distrust remains among patients: 'There's also myth-making in the community, which can make it worse, aunties, mums saying "the implant will make you infertile". Comments like that.'

I told Dr Sowemimo about one piece of surprising data in our poll: 19 per cent of Asian women bought their pills over the counter in pharmacies, compared to 6 per cent of white women,[20] even though contraception is free on the NHS. 'That secrecy. It's not wanting to be seen with contraception among your community. I work in Leicester and it's one of the most diverse cities in the UK, and I know people who travel out of the area to get their contraception. It's why we must do community advocacy work.' Dr Sowemimo also finds 'having greater financial freedom is allowing people to explore private healthcare and thus feel they have greater reproductive autonomy, which many groups previously could not. Yet we're afraid to criticise the system. There's a feeling that people are worried we'll unravel something. There's a hostility to discussion around sexual and repro-ductive health, and the cuts in services means patients are asking for more and we have to deliver on less.'

I got some help with research from the women at GPrX, which provides NHS prescribing data, and it turned out that in 2022 doctors in areas of England with the largest white populations spent four times as much on contra-ception prescriptions than those with the largest ethnic minority populations.[21] Part of that may be personal or religious choice, but it's still a huge gap, and clearly some groups are advocating for themselves more than others. GPrX also found out that the richest areas spent 73 per cent more on contraception than the poorest.

'Part of that is neglect and part could be the misconceptions around reproductive health and ethnic communities, due to outdated patriarchal beliefs,' said Neelam Heera-Shergill, who founded the Cysters charity in Birmingham to combat some of that. Cysters soon became a support group for women too, and Neelam left her job as a lawyer to work there as an advocate and researcher full time. 'We're now a collective changing the current narrative around reproductive well-being, by centring community in our work and ensuring our voices are represented in healthcare fairly,' she said. The impetus came partly from her own experience as a South Asian woman with polycystic ovarian syndrome (PCOS). As an eighteen-year-old student, she was put on the combined pill to help with symptoms. Her doctor (who was South Asian) told her: 'You know that doesn't mean you can go around having sex with everybody.' Neelam explained, 'There's sometimes an assumption in my community that we shouldn't be doing that.'

She said that talking about PCOS, endometriosis and even PMDD is difficult for some women in her community because the use of contraception to help with symptoms is seen as heavily sexualised. 'Doctors are placed on pedestals. We are taught from an early age not a question a doctor as they are always right. There is no room for self-advocacy. There's an imbalance of power. We need to look at women's health strategy through an intersectional lens — there are internal and external barriers to getting the care and contraception we need.' She also said many women are reluctant to take the pill because it's assumed they are sexually promiscuous. 'Virginity is still so prized that the pill is hidden away, or women don't take it at all when it might be needed.' Neelam does a fantastic TEDx talk on YouTube on the myths around virginity.[22] At least we have the choice, even if it is frowned upon in some communities. I'm very aware it's a privilege to be questioning the pill and access, when globally there is desperation around getting contraception at all. In Afghanistan in 2023, the Taliban banned chemists selling any contraceptives to women, claiming their use was a 'Western conspiracy' and 'anti-Muslim'.[23]

I realise that this investigation so far seems tipped against the pill, emphasising the negative rather than positive effects of synthetic hormones, and swinging in the direction of recommending fertility awareness methods. But it's not. I'm coming at this from both sides because I'm also a big fan of what hormones can do. I take natural, body-identical estrogen, progesterone and testosterone every day in my HRT. (And yes, testosterone's a female hormone too; see Chapter 4 on Sex.) I had no idea how important hormones were in the female body and mind until mine all drained away in menopause. I had heart palpitations, joint pain, hot flushes and 4am anxiety, but then I got body-identical HRT, and the symptoms disappeared, I completely recharged, and my memory came flooding back. Previously I'd felt like a clapped-out banger, but now that my hormones are level every day, I feel like I'm motoring steadily at speed, like a Tesla. Wouldn't it be great if more women could feel like that?

For my previous book, *Everything You Need to Know About*

the Menopause (but were too afraid to ask), I investigated the synthetic hormones (conjugated estrogens and the progestin medroxyprogesterone acetate) in the old oral combined forms of HRT, which had been shown to have a small increased risk of breast cancer and clots. I interviewed the world's experts on menopause, and they all agreed that body-identical HRT (transdermal estrogen and natural progesterone) was far safer and better tolerated for most women. Now you may have noticed that synthetic estrogens and progestins are ingredients in the contraceptive pills, and medroxyprogesterone acetate is the progestin in the Depo-Provera contraception injection, so I began to wonder if that could be improved on too, with more body-identical contraceptive pills. There are some newish pills, so far only with body-identical estrogen, but the science is looking good. Why aren't we talking about that, asking for safer pills, and researching new methods and male contraception too? Why has nothing much in the pill recipe changed in sixty years, yet cars have advanced from the three-wheeled Robin Reliant to the Tesla? What on earth are the big pharmaceutical companies doing, apart from raking in billions from their past-the-sell-by-date products?

I'm not a medical doctor – I'm an investigative journalist. I've no vested interest in drugs companies or fertility apps or academic kudos, so I can say what the hell I like and footnote the evidence. I will bring you news of great leaps forward, including the cervical gel which stumps sperm, the temporary jelly vasectomy, and even the Clitoral Doppler Ultrasound. I believe we should understand what is in the pill and how it works. It should be a life skill for every woman, like knowing how to change a tyre. This knowledge is for you, your daughter, or your best friend.

One in four women using contraception in the US or UK take the pill, but this investigation will go beyond that. From that microcosm, a whole world of medical neglect, gender bias and patriarchal control of our bodies begins to be revealed over decades – in history, in science, in economics and in bed. Let's just stop and think about this – how bonkers is it that millions of women who are in perfectly good health go on a drug that gives them side effects for years and may have increased risks of disease in the long term. What's OK about that? Don't we deserve better choices in contraception? And shouldn't this burden be shared with men? I have answers to that further into the book, and some hope for the future. But in the meantime, we need to take control of our hormones – synthetic and natural – before they take control of us.

CHAPTER TWO

CAN WE GO FROM PERIOD
POWER TO PILL POWER?

The grandest family planning clinic I've ever seen was in Park Terrace in Glasgow, a creamy sandstone Victorian townhouse with huge windows, stairs with fancy balustrades, pillars at the entrance and gorgeous views across Kelvingrove Park to the gothic towers of The University of Glasgow. Naturally I was bricking it as I went into that Family Planning Association clinic to get my first contraceptive pill, as a seventeen-year-old law student in my first term. I wouldn't have dared go to my family GP for the pill then, long ago in a time before the iPhone existed, because we didn't mention sex during my Scottish Presbyterian upbringing. It was somehow sinful, slatternly, shameful – and thrilling – to be getting the pill and running off across the park to lose my virginity.

FAKE PERIODS — NO NEED TO BLEED

The Family Planning Association charity went into liqui-dation a few years ago, and that elegant clinic is no longer there with its scary matronly staff and antiseptic smell. Its founding slogan back in 1930 was 'that married people may space or limit their families and thus mitigate the evils of ill health and poverty'. No mention of contraception just for gratuitous shagging. There was also no explanation on my visit to the clinic that it was possible to mitigate the evils of periods by avoiding them altogether on the pill. I suspect the clinic staff had absolutely no idea that it had been known since the advent of the pill that those 21-day green foil packs of Microgynon could be taken non-stop, thus preventing periods altogether.

The bleeds on the combined pill are not periods at all, but fake or 'withdrawal bleeds' caused by the withdrawal of hormones for a week. Somehow, I think we imagined then that if we didn't have a period, menstrual blood would build up inside our wombs until we exploded, but it turns out there is no build-up, just a shedding of the womb lining when the progestin in the pill is stopped for seven days, which is often lighter than the build-up from a normal period. One of the ways hormonal contracep-tives work to prevent pregnancy is by thinning the lining of the womb, the endometrium, which means we also often get lighter periods than we would naturally when we take a pill-free break. This was, unfortunately, not my experience.

MY MOST HUMILIATING PERIOD EVER

After settling down on the pill (twenty-one days on, seven days off), a few years later I found myself writing 'The Freshers' Guide to Contraception' for *Glasgow University Magazine*, researching all the different possibilities from coils to condoms to caps, as well as pills. I remember we no longer included the crab-like Dalkon Shield in the coil photographs, because it had caused horrible pelvic infections and was taken off the market after women sued the manufacturers – see Chapter 6. Even then, I was aware all was not perfect in the contraceptive world. I also got into university politics and became a Students' Representative Council member on the academic governing body, the Senate, which was where my Most Humiliating Period Ever would take place.

I was at some committee in a grand room with gothic windows and a massive table filled with academics, sitting next to an ancient professor who looked like a grey dormouse with glasses. I had elected to wear a longish white circular skirt and a leather jacket that day, and as we were all walking down the grand stairway afterwards, Professor Dormouse came bumbling after me, pointing at the back of my skirt, 'Erm, you seem, um, to have a stain, my dear.' Then he scuttled off. I looked back and there was an enormous, bloody red circle on my white skirt which all the lecturers up the steps behind me could see. I've always been a bit of a flooder. I turned my skirt round, put my bag in front to hide the stain, and ran for the Ladies (in the olden days, there were no gender-neutral toilets at universities). There, I quietly died of embarrassment.

THE 'POPE RULE' FOR PERIODS

Now, had I known I didn't need to have periods at all, that would have been really useful in terms of embarrassment, discomfort and hassle, and would have saved on the cost of roughly three hundred tampons per year. For this we must blame Dr John Rock, the man who played a major role in the development of the birth control pill in the 1950s, and who features in more detail in Chapter 12. Dr Rock, along with Dr Gregory Pincus, conducted the first experiments on American and Puerto Rican women, and they realised early on that the combined pill worked perfectly well when taken non-stop, but decided on a regimen of twenty days on, five days off to reassure new users of this miracle drug that they were not pregnant, and attempt to make the pill seem more 'natural'.

In his 1963 book *The Time Has Come: A Catholic Doctor's Proposals to End the Battle Over Birth Control*, Dr Rock argued that the pill was similar to the church-approved rhythm method, and claimed it completely copied the body's own hormones but just extended the safe period where women would not become pregnant. 'It must be emphasized that the pills, when properly taken, are not at all likely to disturb menstruation,'' he wrote, incorrectly. Dr Rock was keen for the Catholic Church to endorse the pill, as a natural extension of the rhythm method. Pope Paul VI wasn't convinced, and in 1968 put out an encyclical *Humane Vitae* (on human life) confirming the sinfulness of the contraceptive pill. The presence of unnecessary periods became known as 'The Pope Rule'.

IF ONLY SOMEONE HAD TOLD US . . .

I was talking to Hannah Wrathall, who runs a communications agency for women's health and FemTech brands, and who went on the pill at fifteen due to acne and needing birth control for a long-term relationship. I mentioned the fake periods research to her, and she became righteously angry: 'The thing that annoys me most is I used to get really worried when I took two packets back-to-back when I was going on holiday, or to a festival. I thought it might create some weird back-up of my hormones. I now realise that was a really unnecessary worry. I read about the "withdrawal bleeds" somewhere two or three years ago, and honestly it was a lightbulb moment. I can't believe the lies we're told about our own bodies.' Hannah is not alone. In our survey for *Pill Revolution*, 69 per cent of those who took the combined contraceptive pill generally took a monthly seven-day break, and 48 per cent said they did this 'because you have to'.[2]

I first learned about it being safe not to take a break from the pill at the end of Operation Desert Storm in the Gulf War in 1991, when I was embedded as a journalist with the British Army, writing a book about whether women soldiers should go into frontline combat. (Short answer: yes.) It was somewhat gritty living in tents out in the Kuwaiti and Saudi Arabian deserts, but we did have a showering system, which involved standing under a tin bucket of water with holes punched in it, and we also had a long-drop home-dug lavatory. How did the soldiers cope with the mess of periods, and were tampons being delivered with the T-Rats (tinned rations)? I put these questions to a bunch of women truck drivers with the 68 Squadron Royal Corps of Transport. Some of them explained they just took their pill packets back-to-back so periods weren't a problem, and the army doctors concurred.

CONTRACEPTIVE CHOICES AT NUMBER 10 DOWNING STREET

I think those in the know were skipping periods long ago, sometimes as a career decision. Dr Diana Mansour, co-author of the *Contraception Made Easy*[3] textbook, and a consultant in community gynaecology in Newcastle, told me: 'I am in my sixties. I started the pill at the age of twenty or something like that, and I didn't have a period for fifteen years. I remember my mother saying to me that the pill was a revolution for women when I was a medical student, and I thought: I'm not sure this is a huge revolution because even though I'm supposed to be a mother sometime, that's not going to happen. And in those days, you gave your life to the NHS, working a 96-to-120-hour week. Life wasn't easy.'

Some women keep going steady on the pill and have no idea when they roll into menopause. Margaret Thatcher stayed on the pill throughout her reign as prime minister, until she was sixty-three, when she swapped to the hormone replacement therapy (HRT) patch. Teresa Gorman's autobiography *No, Prime Minister!* gives us the lowdown. Shortly after Lady Thatcher was deposed, Gorman had tea with her in Eaton Square and asked her if she used HRT:

'Yes dear, I have a patch,' Mrs Thatcher replied, tapping her bottom as if to indicate that it was in place. 'But I've only had it for eighteen months. You see, no one told me to come off the pill.'

'I was startled. Women usually give up the pill in their fifties, but Margaret was sixty-five [during Gorman's conversation]. "The pill?" I repeated. "Yes," she went on. "You see, Denis and I agreed that I could not risk having more children once I became leader of the party – it was a full-time job. And in those days, I don't think the country was ready for a prime minister on maternity leave. It might have been acceptable in Scandinavia, but not in Britain, at least not when I became leader."[4]

HOW THE PROGESTIN-ONLY AND COMBINED PILL WORK

Back in the early days of the Iron Lady, the main choice was the combined pill, but now it's very different with the increasingly popular progestin-only pill, which is taken non-stop without a break and comes in 28-day packs. It is also called the 'mini-pill' or POP and works by thickening the mucus in the cervix to stop the sperm reaching the egg. The NHS says: 'Your periods may stop or become lighter, irregular or more frequent'[5] on the progestin-only pill, which unhelpfully leaves all possibilities open. The progestin-only pill has to be taken within the same three-hour window every day to prevent pregnancy, unless it contains the progestin desogestrel (brands like Cerelle or Cerazette) and then there's a less stressful twelve-hour window. In our survey,[6] 28 per cent of women got 'spotting between periods' and 11 per cent heavier bleeding on the progestin-only pill, so it looks like you just have to see what form your chaos will take. If you're one of the lucky ones, you may be bleed-free, and this is one of the reasons many trans men and non-binary people like the progestin pill (more of which in Chapter 10).

The combined pill usually contains ethinylestradiol and a progestin, as does the patch and the vaginal ring. You need to take the combined pill at roughly the same time every day and it prevents ovulation and for good measure thickens the mucus in the cervix and thins the lining of the womb, so there is less chance of an egg implanting. With 'correct use' both pills are over 99 per cent effective in preventing pregnancy, but that figure goes down to 91 per cent with normal use. That's where human error and human hangovers come in, as well as sickness or going away for the weekend and forgetting to pack your pill. The useful Contraception Choices website[7] from University College London has a great infographic that shows the failure rate of each method with typical use: the hormonal coil and implant come out top of the class around a 1 per cent pregnancy rate; the progestin injection at 3 per cent; the progestin-only, combined pill and vaginal ring at 9 per cent; the diaphragm at 12 per cent; the male condom at 15 per cent; withdrawal at 22 per cent and fertility awareness at 24 per cent. With no contraception, 85 per cent of women will get pregnant within a year.

IT'S TIME TO START 'TRICYCLING'

But here's a way to help reduce that margin of error and incompetence for the pill – it turns out the 'new' guidance for taking the combined pill is to have a four-day bleed break rather than a seven-day one, or go in for 'tricycling', which is an 84/4 regimen – three months on, four days off – or totally continuous use, 365 days a year.[8] This key advice is highlighted in the seventh edition of the UK text-book *Contraception: Your Questions Answered* by Professors John Guillebaud and Anne MacGregor from 2017,[9] but it still hasn't percolated into the minds of the general public or indeed many doctors prescribing the pill. The book points out that monthly pill-bleeds 'are completely unnecessary for health' and that tricycling is particularly helpful for people with heavy periods. Professor Guillebaud explained that the traditional break is far too long: 'If you take a seven-day break your body starts getting ready to pop out an egg. If you accidentally have an eight-day break you have a high change of ovulating and could therefore get pregnant. To put it another way, a seven-day break gives you very little room for error with remembering to start your new packet.' So, the four-day break, or no break at all, is safer and means you avoid a big crash as your body's regular synthetic hormones are suddenly removed. That crash can cause low mood, bloating, pain, sore breasts, headaches and general misery. For women who are par-ticularly sensitive to changes in hormones, taking the pill non-stop can be much less stressful.

In 2023, Professor Belinda Pletzer of the University of

Salzberg surveyed the mood of 120 women on the pill, and sixty not using contraception, and confirmed what many pill-users had suspected. 'We found that during the pill pause women's mood worsens and they display similar mental health symptoms to those women display during menstruation when they are not on hormonal contraceptives,' she told *Neuroscience News*.[10] Those women who used oral contraceptives showed a 7 per cent increased anxiety score and a 13 per cent increase in negative feelings score during the seven-day pill pause. 'It seems that long-term users, who tolerate their pill well, benefit from mood-stabilizing effects when they are actively taking the pill. In practical terms it may mean that, if women notice a mood worsening during their "pill pause" they should consult with their doctor about adjusting their pill cycles.'

So why oh why has no one bothered to get this healthy and useful message out to women everywhere on the combined pill? Why were seven out of ten women in our survey still taking a seven-day break? Imagine: this advance could reduce heavy faux-periods, hormonal ups and downs, and lower the risk of pregnancy. Professor MacGregor noted dryly in her blog: 'For many women the monthly bleed is an expensive nuisance . . . We hope that manufacturers of the pill will wake up to the twenty-first century and make the pill available for continuous administration, or with a shortened pill-free interval for those women who prefer a monthly "bleed".'[11]

THE FAKE BLEED WAS EMBEDDED INTO PILL
PACKET DESIGN

The fake bleed was engineered into the pill's packaging from the very beginning. Natasha Richardson, who now runs Forage Botanicals providing natural remedies and advice around periods and menopause, did a Masters dissertation at Oxford on the design history of the pill packet and the faux-period. One of the earliest versions in the 1960s was the Ortho DialPak, a pale pink circular plastic box with a ring of twenty-one pills. 'There was very much a commentary at the time on the desirability of the period, taking the pill to be in sync with your period, totally orchestrating your cycle,' said Natasha. The DialPak is in the Smithsonian Museum now.[12] 'It looks like a powder compact, which was easier to secrete in your handbag, and the pill looks white and innocuous, like aspirin.'

One of the very earliest pills was Enovid in 1961, and the American advertisement for that featured a tastefully naked and golden Greek goddess, Andromeda, being freed from her chains, symbolising, of course, the freedom brought by contraception. 'Unfettered', said the title. 'From the beginning, woman has been a vassal to the temporal demands, and frequently the aberrations, of the cyclic mechanism of her reproductive system. Now, to a degree heretofore unknown, she is permitted normalization, enhancement, or suspension of cyclic function and procreative potential.' That did seem to offer 'suspension', but most women knew no better and stuck with the fake bleed.

By 1993, things hadn't improved much, and Americans were offered the Desogen 'Remember Me' Compliance Kit[13] The kit contained pills, a toothbrush, and a bar of soap – and a 'Remember Me' sticker for your bathroom mirror. Text on the pink box bossily ordered women to: 'Brush your teeth, wash your face, take your pill . . . once a day. Every day. At the Same Time.' Desogen had twenty-one white tablets and seven green dummy ones. 'It was a massive sexual revolution – but it was still managed by the patriarchy,' said Natasha. Then, in 2006, came the FDA-approved Seasonique (similar in content to Rigevidon or Microgynon), with one light blue-green tablet for eighty-four consecutive days, followed by one yellow tablet for seven days. It was the first tri-cycle pill. 'The overall design of the pill packet – flamboyant colours, the wallet-like shape, and the frequency of the pills – reflects how the desirability of periods changed over time,' said Natasha.

THE NEW PILLS WITH SHORTER 'BLEEDS'

Interestingly, some of the newer pills containing body-identical natural estrogen have shorter bleeds built in. The combined pill Qlaira has a two-day break, and the levels of estrogen and progestin vary over the month, imitating a natural cycle. 'It's licensed for the treatment of heavy menstrual bleeding as well as contraception,' said Dr Mansour. 'It's a useful option.' Drovelis (or Nextstellis in the US) and Zoely also have body-identical estrogen and a four-day break built in. However, in the UK, because they cost around £8 a month to the NHS (and even more in the US) compared to less than £2 for the older synthetic 21-day versions, prescribing is discouraged, and in many areas of the UK they are unavailable. Don't we deserve better if we're using these pills for years? Answers on a postcard please.

DON'T JUST PUT UP WITH NIGHTMARE PERIODS

I speak here as someone who put up with nightmare periods, without realising they were in fact nightmarishly heavy and long. I just thought they were normal. Particularly after I came off the pill after a few years, my periods got worse, and we all know the joys of bleaching bed sheets and chucking crime-scene knickers in the bin in the toilets and buying an emergency new pair at Marks and Spencer to go back to work. Particularly in my forties in perimenopause (which I wouldn't wish on anyone, but we all go through it), I had unpredictable tsunami periods, requiring two tampons every time I risked a tube journey. I looked up this symptom in science papers, but there wasn't much evidence, so again we had to get our own. In our Channel 4 menopause documentary survey of 4,000 women, 44 per cent said they had extra-heavy periods in perimenopause.[14] Very reassuring after thinking it was just me.

There is a genuine risk when women soldier on with pain or heavy bleeding because it can be a sign of fibroids, endometriosis, adenomyosis or polycystic ovarian syndrome (see Chapter 7), never mind just bad luck, and there are solutions from hormonal coils (see Chapter 6) to the pill-break changes above, and sometimes women need medical intervention. In 2023, the Wellbeing of Women charity launched its 'Just a Period' campaign[15] to highlight the fact that millions of women suffer with severe period pain or heavy bleeding, yet are dismissed and do not get the treatment or support they need. Their testimonies from women were these: 'I'd feel as if my insides were being torn out,' said one. 'I'd cry and scream,' said another. And they continued: 'Sometimes I'd sleep in the bathroom because I'd need to vomit.' 'I just thought it was hereditary.' 'I'd put the tampon in, and I'd get up from the toilet, and literally feel a river's gone whoosh.' What you need to know is that your period should not last more than seven days; interfere with your life; happen more than monthly; need tampon changes more than every two hours; have clots larger than a bottlecap; cause debilitating pain; or make you anaemic. Don't soldier on.

PERIODS TWICE A MONTH?

What if you have a period twice a month? When Lauren Chiren was a teenager, she had twenty-one periods a year, coming every fifteen to sixteen days. 'I didn't know any different. I was doing lots of sport, and it was also very light,' she said. But her hormones were haywire. 'From aged eleven to sixteen, I had to work really hard at controlling my temper. I had the shortest fuse on the planet for half the month. I'm a Scottish redhead and blew my fuse at the slightest thing.' Going on the combined pill was a lifesaver. 'The pill gave me a sense of control and calm, and I didn't come off it until I started trying to get pregnant in my thirties.' A few years after she had her son, she was back on the pill and was seriously injured doing judo, and eventually realised she was actually post-menopausal in her early forties. Lauren now lives in Bristol, training menopause coaches and champions internationally to support executives going through menopause. 'If you're not experiencing bleeding on the pill, it's hard to know what it is doing to your body over the long term,' she said. 'I wish I'd known that I was in menopause and could have taken hormone replacement therapy earlier.' The *Pill Revolution* poll showed that aside from preventing pregnancy, 48 per cent were using it to regulate or lessen periods, 13 per cent to control acne, 9 per cent to help with conditions like polycystic ovarian syndrome and endometriosis, and 8 per cent to help with premenstrual syndrome.[16]

FROM PERIOD POWER TO PILL POWER

There's been much talk in the last decade about Period Power — embracing the forces of your menstrual cycle, ending shame around periods, and increasing knowledge — along with the movement led by younger people to try to end period poverty and improve access to sanitary products. There have been so many books written about understanding your menstrual cycle and taking control of your activities, changing diet and exercise, including Maisie Hill's valuable *Period Power*.[17] But where is the Pill Power movement? When will we arm ourselves with knowledge to make informed choices, and demand better and safer forms of contraception for women and men?

THE MENSTRUAL CYCLE — FOLLICLES, FIREWORKS AND FLATLINING

Let's open our laywoman's toolbox and understand how hormones work during the natural menstrual cycle – and how synthetic hormones can have very different effects. We learned about the four stages of the menstrual cycle at school – period, follicular phase, ovulation, luteal phase – but when starting to research this book, I certainly needed a recap. Starting from day one of your period, the first half of the cycle – leading up to the ovulation mountain of estrogen – is known as the follicular phase, and generally women feel energetic, as estrogen levels pump up. Then, a day or so before ovulation, in comes the follicle-stimulating hormone (FSH), which releases the most-developed follicle (a bag of fluid containing a developing egg), hoping for impregnation. Then the fireworks go off, desire rockets, and ovulation occurs mid-month as the follicle bursts open and the egg is released to freedom down the fallopian tubes. Next, enter the luteinising hormone (LH), which signals to the remains of the follicle, now an empty shell known as the corpus luteum, to release progesterone. Progesterone peaks at around day twenty-two and then crashes, along with estrogen, as the period looms again and our hormones flatline.

WHAT'S MISSING FROM THE PICTURE?
TESTOSTERONE

Which female hormone is missing from all these monthly menstrual diagrams in Wikipedia, Britannica, Women's Health Network and the school GCSE biology exam notes? Testosterone. In perhaps one of the worst gender biases yet to be overturned in medicine, testosterone is often still considered to be a male-only sex hormone, when in fact it is gender neutral. Women make about a tenth of the amount testosterone men do, mostly in their ovaries, and it generally stays steady, with a small but joyous leap in the middle of the month at the time of ovulation. Women's brains are full of testosterone receptors, and as you might expect there are plenty more around the vulva, vagina and clitoris. But testosterone is about so much more than sex. For women and men it has a positive effect on energy, motivation, memory, muscle mass and bone density. Testosterone matters. Later on, we will talk about the effect of high testosterone in women with polycystic ovarian syndrome, and the fact that the progestins in hormonal contraception increase sex hormone binding globulin, which basically binds or ties up the estrogen and testosterone in your body, and therefore lowers the free circulating testosterone available to women. Professor Nick Panay, a consultant gynaecologist at Imperial College in London and president of the International Menopause Society, noted as far back as 2006 that 'young women's ovaries produce approximately three to four times more testosterone than estrogen daily'[18] Testosterone is women's most biologically active hormone, and although it declines steadily from your early twenties onwards, it's the last hormone left standing (at least in small quantities) after the age of fifty-one, when progesterone and estrogen disappear at menopause.

PREMENSTRUAL SYNDROME

There are volumes of literature dedicated to premenstrual syndrome (PMS), the result of our hormonal rollercoaster when progesterone and estrogen slump before a period, but we'll cover the basics here. The NHS says: 'PMS is a recurring pattern of emotional, physical and behavioural changes in the days before your period that impact your daily life . . . mood swings, feeling upset, anxious or irritable, tiredness or trouble sleeping, bloating or tummy pain, breast tenderness, headaches, spotty skin, greasy hair, changes in appetite and sex drive.'[19] Unfortunately, the NHS description is a bit bland. In fact, we all have our own special version of PMS, and this was mine: 'Low, vicious mood. Slept under desk at work. Want to kill boyfriend for crunching crisps at 100 decibels. Top button popped on trousers. Am I pregnant or just BLOATING LIKE A BALLOON? Breasts have rocks in them. Hair is dripping like a chip shop, even though I washed it today. Huge subterranean evil spot. Ate six-pack of Tunnocks' teacakes, only 106 calories each, still feel sick.' That's PMS. For some women, the pill can stop the descent into darkness by keeping hormones steady, if slightly lower than the natural version, and for those who are extra-sensitive to hormonal fluctuations, avoiding pill breaks altogether can be helpful.

Dr Katharina Dalton, patron saint of PMS

Interestingly, Dr Katharina Dalton, who coined the term PMS in a *British Medical Journal* study in 1953, was trying to treat women with top-up hormones right from the start, but she believed in using natural body-identical progesterone rather than synthetic progestins. She worked with endocrinologist Dr Raymond Greene (who happened to be brother of novelist Graham Greene). Dr Dalton opened the world's first PMS clinic at University College Hospital in London, after experiencing the disappearance of her monthly migraines while she was pregnant, which alerted her to the fact the headaches were affected by low progesterone levels. She invented the phrase premenstrual syndrome and explained it was a cyclical illness that starts after ovulation, with the most severe symptoms appearing in the final four days before menstruation. She used menstrual charts to diagnose the disorder, and argued that PMS in women could explain higher rates of suicide attempts, alcohol abuse and violent crimes around that time. She appeared as an expert witness to explain this in court. She was part of the successful mitigation in two famous cases: that of Anna Reynolds, who killed her mother while suffering from postnatal depression, and Nicola Owen, an arsonist who set fire to homes in Richmond and Twickenham, in London, at intervals which were multiples of twenty-eight days.

PREMENSTRUAL DYSPHORIC DISORDER

Some of the conditions Dr Dalton was treating would now be described as premenstrual dysphoric disorder (PMDD), which is much more severe than PMS, and often lasts for the whole of the luteal phase after ovulation. The mental health effects can include suicidal feelings, anxiety and depression, and many people find it interferes with functioning at work and in relationships. The menstrual hormone changes may cause a serotonin deficiency, which can affect mood. Some doctors prescribe antidepressants, selective serotonin reuptake inhibitors (SSRI), which can be taken for all or just part of the month. It's peculiar, though, that very few professionals consider the option of just topping up those natural falling hormones, and we discuss that later in the book.

Dr Dalton argued that premenstrual mood changes were brought on primarily by deficiencies of progesterone and could be improved by taking natural progesterone pessaries, and even suggested that post-natal depression could also be treated with progesterone. (In fact, in the seventy years since Dr Dalton came up with the idea of hormonal top-ups, there have been a number of studies showing that taking body-identical progesterone,[20] as well as transdermal estrogen after pregnancy can help prevent the baby blues.) Where would billions of women round the world be without the work of Dr Dalton? Where is her Nobel Prize? Since it will be twenty years since her death in September 2024, I'm going to work on a campaign for an English Heritage blue plaque to go up on the wall of

University College Hospital, on behalf of all the women who have been helped by her identification of PMS. Watch this space.

PROGESTINS — HOW THEY WORK IN MYSTERIOUS WAYS

Dr Dalton refused to use synthetic progestins in her work, as she believed they were the cause of side effects, and she pointed out that only natural progesterone fitted the progesterone receptors in the body and the brain. How prescient she was, back in the 1950s and 1960s, when the contraceptive pill was just coming into wider circulation. Let's crunch into how progestins and their receptors work in more detail, because it can change how each brand of pill or contraception affects you personally. A hormone receptor is a protein that binds hormones. Once the hormone receptor and the hormone are bound together, it starts a cascade of actions in the body or the mind. But synthetic progestins are not always derived from progesterone. Instead, many progestins are derived from testosterone, and one, drospirenone, from the diuretic drug spironolactone. The shape of a molecule of progestin is different from the shape of a molecule of natural progesterone, and the synthetic progestin can go rogue and hook up with other unrelated receptors – the androgen receptor, the estrogen receptor and the glucocorticoid steroid receptor. And nobody seems to know exactly what's going on[21] – least of all you and your body. The interaction might be positive, negative or just have no effect at all. But what we have learned, by trial and much error on women, is that the different progestins in different pills can have profound effects on health, and reading the label on a packet and identifying which group your progestin is in may have life-improving results.

Myth-busting progestins

The progestins derived from testosterone have, as you might expect, a more androgenic effect on women. These pills may work well for you, but they can also cause acne, unwanted body and facial hair, vaginal dryness, low mood, low libido, breast tenderness, headaches and PMS. If a particular pill is giving you side effects, you might want to switch to a pill with lower progestin, a less-androgenic progestin, or a higher estrogen pill, which could also help with any breakthrough bleeding. If your combined pill seems too estrogenic, you could have side effects like pain from breast fullness, migraines, bloating, nausea, tiredness, irritability, fluid retention and weight gain, so it might be worth changing the quantity of estrogen or going on a progestin-only pill.

So here's a list of some progestins and their possible effects. Think of it as learning a new, useful language – Duolingo for contraception. I won't name all the specific pills, as many have the same ingredients. For instance, Microgynon, Rigivedon and Seasonale all have the same testosterone-derived progestin in them, levonorgestrel, as does the hormonal coil, but in a much lower dose. But you can check out your pill contents at www.medicines. org.uk, and The Lowdown website and the Clue app[22] are also helpful on this.

THE DIFFERENT KINDS OF PROGESTINS

Androgenic progestins

- Progestins derived from testosterone include: levonorgestrel, norgestrel and gestodene. Norethindrone, norethindrone acetate and ethynodiol diacetate are slightly less androgenic.

- Newer progestins like norgestimate and desogestrel have little or no androgenic activity.

- Medroxyprogesterone acetate is derived from progesterone, but still has some androgenic effects.

- The morning-after pill, brands like Levonelle in the UK, or Plan B in the US, contain a much larger dose of levonorgestrel than the daily pill, but the progestin only remains in your body for a short time. Other pills like ellaOne contain the progesterone receptor modulator ulipristal acetate.

Anti-androgenic progestins

- Anti-androgenic progestins derived from progesterone include: chlormadinone acetate, cyproterone acetate and dienogest.

- Drospirenone is also anti-androgenic, and derived from spironolactone.

- The new generation of pills with body-identical estrogen still have synthetic progestins in them. Zoely has nomegestrol acetate, which has some anti-androgenic activity, Qlaira has dienogest and Drovelis has drospirenone.

WHICH PILL?

It looks hellishly complicated, but the above list will help you detect which type of pill you already have, and you could just ask your doctor to swap your pill for something more androgenic or estrogenic, depending on your symptoms. The problem is that each pill affects each woman differently, and reactions are hard to predict. As Dr Sally Darnborough, a GP and women's health specialist working in Argyll and the islands told me: 'I sometimes feel like an alchemist working out what each woman needs. We usually start with Rigevidon or Microgynon in a healthy young person, it's a basic combined starter pill. It's been around the longest and has the most evidence for safety. But if women have existing problems with skin, facial hair and PMS, I might prescribe Yasmin, Dianette or similar. I'm prescribing the pill, Depo-Provera and implants less, as more women request IUDs [coils] for convenience and better bleeding control.' Dr Darnborough recommended the Faculty of Sexual and Reproductive Healthcare website[23] as a really detailed source on this for doctors and patients. She explained that lots of pills, like the new ones with body-identical estrogen, are not always listed on the local formulary or prescribing list due to cost restrictions. But so long as they are on the NHS British National Formulary, doctors can issue them. 'We've had supply issues which have influenced prescribing. I'm not a maverick prescriber, but I'll offer an alternative within FRSH guidance. It makes sense to find something better if young girls might stop the pill due to side effects and get pregnant.'

WHY DON'T WE LEARN ABOUT THE PILL AT SCHOOL?

Understanding that the pill exists in dozens of different versions, with opposite effects, and can be changed to suit you, would have been a great thing to learn in school. I was talking to an eighteen-year-old who had just made aspirin from scratch in his lab in A-level Chemistry. Why can't we teach pupils the basics about the contraceptive pill too? Knowing the estrogenic or androgenic effects of each pill could also be helpful for trans and non-binary people, who are looking to marginally alter their hormone balance, or use contraception that works alongside gender-affirming hormones.

GENDER-DIVERSE CONTRACEPTION NEEDS

On that note, I want to welcome readers of any gender identity. The nature of this book, which deals largely with the results and risks of cisgender heterosexual sex, means I am mostly using 'woman' to mean someone who has ovaries and a womb and can get pregnant, but that can include some trans men and non-binary people too. When I say 'men', I suppose I mean people with penises, which sounds rather mechanistic, and that can include some trans women and non-binary people. In Chapter 10, I investigate the trans, non-binary and gender-queer contraceptive experience more fully with an expert. Anyway, you all know exactly who you are, and I hope you, your womb and your brain will feel included, and that your experience will be reflected somewhere in these pages. I'd also like to hear more from you for future work because the academic research is simply not there yet.

SIDE EFFECTS MATTER

As I noted earlier, 77 per cent of women experience side effects on hormonal contraception, and now that we know about the masculinising and feminising effects of different progestins, and the weird fact that they can hook up with estrogen and testosterone receptors too, is it any wonder that the pill exerts so many changes beyond just stopping conception? And even if those side effects are only serious for 10 per cent of women, those women really matter and should not be gaslighted. While we still sometimes blame ourselves for symptoms, the physical evidence of the effect of the pill is there – the suppression of estrogen production 'is profound and clearly visible by ultrasound where oral contraception use may halve the size of the ovaries,'[24] and added synthetic hormones only replace our natural hormones to some extent. In contrast, the progestin exposure in about half the brands of pills can be four times our natural levels of progesterone.[25] There's a lot of action there – no wonder we have a reaction.

WEIGHT GAIN

There are many very serious side effects of the pill, and I discuss mental health, blood clots, breast cancer risk, lowered libido and brain changes in separate chapters. But the side effect women complained of most in our survey was weight gain, which affected 37 per cent. Now there are lots of caveats here and other reasons for weight gain, which is sometimes unfairly blamed on the pill. In fact, 59 per cent of women in the UK are overweight, and 69 per cent in the US,[26] and teenage girls naturally put on weight in puberty as breasts and hips grow, often at the same time they start the pill. So, what do the websites say? On the Planned Parenthood website, it says: 'Some people think that the hormones in the pill cause weight gain or weight loss, but that's not true.'[27] On the NHS website, it says: 'There is no evidence that the pill will make you gain weight.'[28] Both those official statements are questionable, but no one would go near the pill if it stated in black and white – 'Let's be honest, this may cause you to gain a couple of pounds'. It would be a PR disaster for contraception. Although it's a complicated picture when it comes to weight gain, women know their own truth, as we saw in the survey, and if they are already questioning the link between weight gain and hormonal birth control, why shouldn't they deserve to know what the science says?

Ben and Jerry's in the luteal phase

We already know that natural hormones affect eating habits across the menstrual cycle. Women tend to eat less during the first follicular phase, and more during the later luteal phase heading into PMS, when we scarf down a whole tub of Ben and Jerry's Cookie Dough while watching Netflix. In the follicular phase, higher levels of estrogen increase satiating hormones in the stomach, and there is also a decrease in preference for sweet foods. But when women are on combined pills, they make more sex hormone binding globulin, which lowers free testosterone. Low testosterone can cause weight gain, then excess body fat produces more estrogen, which starts a vicious circle lowering testosterone again. With periods starting on average at twelve years old, and increasingly even younger, coupled with the increasing use of the pill to reduce periods, there is a chance that girls' endocrine systems get disrupted at a young age and this could increase the risk of weight gain.

An overview of the science on weight gain

The Cochrane Database, which is one of the most reliable sources of medical research, looked at twenty-two studies of 11,450 women in total on whether oral contraceptives caused weight gain,[29] and concluded that mean weight gain at six or fourteen months was less than 2kg (4.4lb) for most studies, and this was similar to people using other forms of birth control. They said many of the data available was of a low standard and did not come from randomised controlled trials. Two studies showed a greater increase in body fat for users of hormonal coils versus women not using a hormonal method. One also showed a similar difference with a progestin-only pill, and two studies showed a greater decrease in lean body mass with progestin-only contraception use.

A review of fifteen studies looking at the effects of progestin-only contraceptives on weight, showed that twelve did not detect any changes, but three studies did find gains of an average of 2kg a year.[30] So it's not entirely clear. But there's definitely proven weight gain among users of the Depo-Provera medroxyprogesterone contraceptive injections, and one study showed that adolescents had a greater increase in body fat than older women. Even the NHS admits this one, explaining that with the injection 'weight gain is often less than 4lbs (2.2kg) over one to two years, but it can sometimes be up to 8lbs (4.4kg).[31]

From size 6 to 12 in a few months

That's the science, such as it is, but what's the human experience? What if you are one of the small group of women whose hormones go haywire on the pill, causing unexpected weight gain? Eloise Donovan, now twenty-six, works in investment banking in London, and believes taking the combined pill at an early age rocked her metabolism. 'I was skinny and small when I got my period for the first time at thirteen and found that I was bleeding constantly for seven weeks at a time. I probably had anaemia. About eight months later, my mum took me to the doctor and I went on Microgynon, and no one told me about any possible side effects. I went from a size 6 to 8 to 12 in a few months. It happened so fast I got thick red stretch red marks all down my legs and hips.' The marks made Eloise ashamed to go swimming, and she was keen on sport and enjoyed playing netball too. 'A gynaecologist was quite firm and said "the pill can't make you put on weight" but it's rubbish – I definitely wasn't unhealthy. This gaslighting of women is a huge thing.' Actually, the small print in the Microgynon patient leaflet in the pill box says: 'Common side effects (between 100 and 1,000 in every 10,000 users may be affected): feeling sick, stomach ache, putting on weight, headaches, depressive moods or mood swings, sore or painful breasts.'[32] But I never read that leaflet when I went on Microgynon, and neither did Eloise when she was fourteen.

'Teenagers have nowhere to channel this'

Feeling fat made Eloise depressed, and she says this was a defining time for her mental health. 'I was basically starving myself, and I didn't go on holiday because I didn't want anyone to see me.' Eventually, she changed her pill to Yasmin, but no one ever suggested she should stop or take a break for a while and see if her periods were working normally. 'I wasn't sexually active then. I was just too terrified *not* to be on this pill.' Then aged twenty-one, she came off the pill, and her clothes size came down to size 8 to 10 and her moods improved. 'I was still so conscious of my red stretch marks I got them zapped with a laser so now they are silver, but you can still see them.' She also had some therapy afterwards. 'I was such a happy child until that point, and I am happy now, but I was very unhappy then. My mum is still upset with herself that she didn't question it all. Teenagers have nowhere to channel this into. When you're fourteen years old you don't even have a voice.'

WHERE ARE THE BODY-IDENTICAL HORMONES FOR YOUNGER WOMEN?

I investigate more about the effects of synthetic hormones on the changing bodies and brains of adolescents in Chapter 5. But as someone who uses body-identical transdermal estrogen and testosterone, plus oral progesterone as hormone replacement therapy, and is thankful daily for its positive effects on my brain, metabolism and energy, I wondered: why are we still wedded to putting synthetic hormones into younger women, when the 'gold standard' in HRT is body-identical hormones, recommended by the International Menopause Society? The science isn't quite there yet on all fronts, and synthetic progestins are more powerful than progesterone. But why are older women in menopause able to choose better, safer hormones, while younger ones are being left behind?

A MINI 'CHEMICAL MENOPAUSE' ON SOME PROGESTIN-ONLY CONTRACEPTION?

Dr Louise Newson runs the largest menopause clinic in the world from Stratford-upon-Avon in England, as well as a non-profit research arm, and is an adviser on the government menopause taskforce. I worked with her on my menopause book, and helped her set up The Menopause Charity. She often sends me a thrilling scientific paper at midnight and has an extraordinary ability to think out of the box. Her research into the very different behaviour of synthetic and natural body-identical hormone replacement in menopausal women has also led her to look more closely at the synthetic hormones used on millions of younger women – including her own daughters.

'Synthetic hormones are associated with more risks, albeit small ones, compared to body-identical hormones, including a small risk of clot and possibly breast cancer,' said Dr Newson. 'When younger women are given contraceptives that contain synthetic hormones, they often stop egg production, and therefore work as a contraception.' The combined pill completely stops ovulation, and the progestin-only pill stops ovulation in around 60 per cent of women, while the rest may continue to ovulate – it's unpredictable and inconsistent.'[33] 'What so many people don't realise is that when women don't produce eggs, it also means that the associated hormones associated with the egg production are reduced. Women who use progestin-only contraception, for example implants, are essentially given a chemical menopause, meaning that they will have low estrogen and testosterone levels in their bodies. This can result in symptoms like low mood, memory problems, reduced libido, anxiety, weight gain and joint pains.'

Some studies have also shown that the 'mini-menopause' from progestin-only contraceptives can be linked to a reduction in bone density, also related to the low hormone levels. Adolescents starting the pill early on seem to be more at risk than older women,[34] and the Royal Osteoporosis Society says that the Depo-Provera progestin contraceptive injection can lower bone density. Dr Newson explained that the combined contraceptive pill might be better, 'because it does contain a synthetic estrogen which has some bone-protective effects, although that's less than the body-identical transdermal estrogen we prescribe on HRT. However, oral estrogen increases sex hormone binding globulin, which leads to a reduction in bioavailable testosterone in the body. When women have reduced testosterone, this can reduce libido and it can also affect mood, energy and concentration.'

A SCANDALOUS LACK OF RESEARCH

Again and again, the message keeps coming through: don't struggle on if you are suffering. Consider changing to a different brand or method of contraception for a while, and track how it affects your mental and physical health before and after. Trust in your own feelings. Take Pill Power into your own hands. Dr Newson said: 'We are all individuals, and should make decisions regarding contraception choices based on individual risks and benefits. I'm sure going forwards that many younger women will choose the low-dose progestin coils for contraception, and if they need hormones, for example to improve PMS symptoms, then they'll elect to have body-identical hormones to stabilise their estradiol [estrogen] levels and replace low testosterone as appropriate.' She finishes with a powerful point: 'It's scandalous and barbaric that so little research has been done into women's hormones and the biological effects of stopping our natural hormones by giving us contraception.'

CHAPTER THREE

HOW DOES THE PILL AFFECT YOUR MENTAL HEALTH?

'The pill picked at me a little bit every day. I lost something.'

Those are the words of Kirsty Keating, who went on hormonal contraception at fourteen, and only discovered when she came off the pill permanently at thirty that it had been turning her into a different person. We will hear more from Kirsty later, but her experience shows that there is a humungous gap between some women's gruelling experience of mental health problems while on the pill, and the medical establishment's much cheerier version of the situation.

In a poll we conducted of 4,000 women for our *Pill Revolution* documentary, an astonishing 57 per cent said they worried about the possible effect of hormonal contraception on their mental health.[1] Yet Planned Parenthood makes no mention whatsoever of mental health side effects in its basic contraceptive pill guide[2] for Americans, although headaches, sore breasts and nausea do make the cut. In the UK, the NHS website advises the combined pill 'can cause temporary side effects at first, such as . . . mood swings – if these do not go after a few months, it may help to change to a different pill.'[3] There's similar advice on the progestin-only pill. No problem, women think, popping their first pill. Just a wee mood swing . . .

WHY IS OUR REAL EXPERIENCE OF DEPRESSION ON THE PILL IGNORED?

Of course, Planned Parenthood and the NHS want women and people with ovaries who are having sex to use contraception, for very sensible reasons, and anything that makes patients question their initial decision is played down in official advice. For the majority of women, the pill is a perfectly safe form of birth control and goes down a treat. It stops or lessens periods and often steadies mood when previously women might have had debilitating premenstrual syndrome (PMS). When the pill is good, it is very, very good – but when it's bad, it's appalling. This is not sufficiently acknowledged, so people cannot make a fully informed decision to choose the pill – or stay on it.

Thanks to the official downplaying of this risk, individual women fail to see themselves clearly. They fail to recognise and question their own symptoms and changes to their behaviour. They blame themselves, not the pill. As the pioneering Australian psychiatrist and hormone expert Professor Jayashri Kulkarni told me: 'Basic neuroscience tells us that the hormones estrogen, testosterone and progesterone are potent brain steroids,' and everyone should understand that the synthetic hormones in the pill can have as profound effect on the mind as they do so on the reproductive system. 'There's not a stainless-steel plate at waist level which stops hormones getting up to our heads,' she added.

So 'mood swings' are real, but that vague term can disguise a grimmer truth. 'Swing' sounds as if it might mean up as well as down. For dozens of women who have shared their experiences with me, the only direction was down – to depression, emotional numbness, fatigue, severe anxiety, and for a rare few, suicidal thoughts. In our *Pill Revolution* survey, 36 per cent said they had experienced depression, anxiety or low mood on hormonal contraception and over a third of women told us they came off the pill for mental health reasons. That's women's truth, but it's not what you'll read in the medical textbooks.

Later in this chapter, I'll unpack the major pieces of scientific research on depression, anxiety and hormonal contraception, and look particularly at the added risks for vulnerable adolescents, who are often prescribed the pill early just to prevent acne or lessen period pain. But for now, I want to tell you more about Kirsty Keating, from Tring, Hertfordshire, who went on the combined pill as a teenager and stayed on it for years. It set her life on a completely different path.

'At fourteen years old I had terrible acne on my back, chest and face. I'd tried all the topical treatments, and they didn't work, so I was then prescribed Dianette. It was great. It was a big change, massive for me.' (The combined pill Dianette contains the progestin cyproterone acetate and a high dose of synthetic estrogen.) 'It clamps down on all the male hormones,' said Kirsty. Dianette certainly does – that particular progestin is an anti-androgen, so it reduces testosterone, which can cause acne, and also boosts estrogen. But as I've explained before, female testosterone also helps with energy, muscle building, mental sharpness and drive, so shutting that down along with the pimples is an important side effect women are not told about.

'It did get rid of my acne at the time, but I'd been a very sparky blonde, in-your-face Gemini, and suddenly I was coming up to my mock exams, and I wasn't going to school. I couldn't do my GCSEs. I just couldn't go. No one ever asked why – they thought it was just teenage mood stuff. I pulled out of school.' There were other changes. Kirsty lost her sex drive completely thanks to the lack of testosterone. 'There was literally nothing,' she said. The Dianette patient leaflet says: 'Uncommon side effects (may affect up to 1 in 100 people) . . . loss of interest in sex,' and that 'Common side effects (may affect up to 1 in 10 people) . . . putting on weight.'[4] Kirsty also put on a lot of weight and suffered an eating disorder. That might not be a side effect of the pill, but Kirsty suspects so, all part of a bigger picture of decline. 'It was like it picked at you a little bit every day. I lost something.'

But like many of us, Kirsty blamed herself for the changes, and never read the words in the Dianette leaflet which say: 'Psychiatric disorders: Some women using hormonal contraceptives including Dianette have reported depression or depressed mood. Depression can be serious and may sometimes lead to suicidal thoughts. If you experience mood changes and depressive symptoms contact your doctor for further medical advice as soon as possible.'[5] By the time Kirsty was twenty-one, she was still on Dianette. 'I was very, very unwell, agoraphobic and housebound. I got lots of psychotherapy and no one ever asked about hormones.' But she accidentally got pregnant and sadly lost the baby, and that changed things. 'I realised I'd like to start a family.' She stopped taking the pill, cleared her body of synthetic hormones, and her life went into turnaround. 'I set up my own cleaning business within six months. I had energy again.' With her husband, she had her first son at twenty-two. She went on to have a second son, and by the age of thirty, doctors started her on the progestin-only pill. 'I went on the mini-pill, and it spun my world upside down, I felt physically terrible and mentally clouded, yet again feeling that I couldn't and didn't want to do day-to-day things. My GP wanted to put me on antidepressants. I knew this wasn't right for me. I wasn't depressed, my life was happy and stable.' Luckily, this time her husband was on the lookout and noticed the patterns. He told Kirsty: 'When you hit thirty, you literally changed. You stopped speaking and you didn't want to go out.' They discussed together whether it was the pill, and Kirsty came off it. 'It was a eureka moment!' She felt so much better without hormonal contraception. 'He gave me a massive hug and said he'd get a vasectomy.'

Kirsty is now forty-four, with sons aged sixteen and twenty-one. She has had ten happy years without hormonal contraception and is now in early menopause. 'I'm a huge advocate for early menopause now I'm on that journey, and I'm encouraging my friends to have their hormone levels tested. I'm very loud now, very aware of hormones. I could have spotted things earlier and made connections sooner. We need to look after the next generation.'

STARTING YOUNG

On that note, it seems the next generation may be in peril. In our survey, 64 per cent of pill-users in the UK went on it aged eighteen or under, and almost a fifth of those were girls aged fifteen or less. Schoolkids are making this major life decision, and I suspect they and their parents are not as well informed as they think – either by videos on TikTok or a hurried, tick-tocking nine-minute slot with their GP. Like Kirsty, many start the pill for non-contraceptive reasons: 13 per cent use it to improve acne and 48 per cent to improve periods. But while spots and period pain are often vanquished, we discovered in our survey that there might be a cost: rates of low mood, anxiety and depression were much higher in the 16–24 age group, at 55 per cent.

Of course, puberty's crazy anyway with hormones all over the shop, so the pill should by no means take the blame for everything. But synthetic hormones have a powerful effect, good and bad, on the half-cooked adolescent brain, which is busy pruning old connections and strengthening new ones. It's particularly discombobulating for a teenager already at risk of depression. During adolescence, puberty is kick-started by the hypothalamic-pituitary-gonadal axis, which causes a huge release of estrogen, testosterone and progesterone that leads to sexual maturity, while the brain is being completely remodelled. Do the natural and synthetic hormones work in tandem? And what about the unnaturally high doses of progestins in certain pills?[6] We just don't know enough about how replacing natural hormones with synthetic ones affects the growth of the brain — yet.

THE NEW SCIENCE ON MOOD AND HORMONAL CONTRACEPTION

The Faculty of Sexual Health and Reproductive Healthcare (FSRH) is the leading UK body for medical professionals on birth control. It has a super-accurate website,[7] with levels of clinical evidence assessed, and it also tests and reviews the latest contraceptives. I use it a lot to double-check contraception facts. So, the FSRH's opinion on the possible link between mood disorders and the pill is weighty. The problem is there have been very few randomised controlled trials (RCTs), in which two separate similar groups are randomly given a drug, or a placebo, and monitored over time. This is considered the scientific 'gold standard', but it isn't easy with contraception, since in some cases testers might have to use condoms, not knowing whether they were on the pill or not. There's little enthusiasm from participants for such trials, and they are expensive. Plus, the major research funders, generally pharmaceutical companies, have no incentive to go around testing to find out whether their own best-selling products have deleterious effects on mental health.

This means that observational studies, paid for by academic institutions, are the best option. These studies look at large population-tracking health databases, which show the different trajectories of women on or off the pill. The FSRH analysed around twenty research papers on mood and contraception, giving more weight to RCTs than observational studies. Thus, their clinical guidelines say: 'the available evidence does not establish a causal relationship' between progestin pills and depression[8] and that 'the evidence suggests that some women may experience negative mood changes when taking combined hormonal contraception. However, there is not clear, consistent evidence that combined hormonal contraception use causes depression; mood change is common and often related to external events.'[9]

I'd beg to differ from that opinion – strongly. The FSRH and the medical establishment need to err on the side of caution and weigh up the evidence with that in mind. But I'm on the side of radical enquiry, and the FSRH only looked at research up until 2018. Since those guidelines came out, there have been a number of pieces of fascinating new research and neuroscience which I'd like to draw to your attention.

Most of the major critical thinking on contraception – and its link to mental health – is coming out of Scandinavian universities and hospitals, which are able to get public funding for large-scale studies. The Nordic countries also have high-quality contraceptive counselling, and one of the lowest abortion rates in the world: 11 per 1,000 women aged 15–49[10] compared to 19 per 1,000 in the UK. They're doing something right, and that's perhaps why they're not afraid to question the perfect-pill orthodoxy.

The grandfather of the movement is Professor Øjvind Lidegaard in the Obstetrics and Gynaecology department at Copenhagen University. He has completed major investigations in this area, including charting the likelihood of clots and breast cancer risk depending on contraception type. His former PhD student, Dr Charlotte Wessel Skovlund, dug into the vast Danish medical database and tracked what happened to the mental health of over one million women aged fifteen to thirty-four on hormonal contraception (without prior depression diagnosis) over six years.[11] The results were published in 2016 in the *Journal of the American Medical Association*, and it turned out users of the progestin-only pill were 34 per cent more likely to be prescribed antidepressants, and combined pill-users had an increase of 23 per cent.

Those on the hormonal coil were 40 per cent more likely to get antidepressants, and levels were even higher for those using the vaginal ring and patch. Among adolescents, the results were more worrying: those on the progestin-only pill were 120 per cent more likely to get a first prescription of antidepressants, and there was an 80 per cent increase with the combined pill. Dr Skovlund said, 'There was a huge reaction in the media to our findings.' But in the UK, the FSRH concluded that 'significant confounding factors cannot be excluded, and a causative association is not established' and pointed to other major studies across the world which had not shown the contraception–depression link.[12] It's certainly possible to theorise that the Danish self-selecting hormonal contraception users were more likely to be moody and sexually active – but on this million-woman scale?

I got on a Zoom call with Professor Lidegaard and put these concerns to him. He pointed out that other large studies of the side effects experienced by women on the pill often remove those sensitive to depression beforehand. 'Other studies follow women who are happy on the pill and not those who give up on it. Our big observational study gives real-life data. Depression risk goes up for women generally on hormonal contraception, and in the fifteen to nineteen age group it's double the rate.'

He is not against hormonal contraception as such, which works for so many. 'The majority of women are fine on the pill, so no one pays much attention to the minority. We didn't conduct these studies to scare people away, but to make them wiser and provide them with a basis on which they can decide whether the benefits of taking this product outweigh the risks. We need to understand that women have very different reactions to the same products, and the minority shoulder very severe changes in their mood. Some of them even develop depression within a few weeks after starting use. Many of them are not aware that these products could have a responsibility for the changes and then continue to use them unquestioning as they go into severe depression.' Professor Lidegaard had a suggestion: 'We need to take better histories when prescribing contraceptives, particularly from younger women. Have they previously had depression, hormonal mood swings, problems?'

After completing the research with Professor Lidegaard in 2016, Dr Skovland thought there would be an upsurge in research on contraception and mental health. 'I kind of expected that there would a lot of new investigations into this area afterwards, but I don't think there has been that much. Actually, that's interesting in itself . . . ' She shrugged. Dr Skovlund followed up with another investigation into almost half a million young women with the average age of twenty-one in the same Danish database and found that starting the pill doubled their risk of a first suicide attempt, compared with non-users of hormonal contraceptives. 'In Denmark anyway, it's like the normal thing to do is to get the pill and get your first boyfriend. Your mother probably goes with you to the doctor,' Dr Skovlund told me. (Like everyone I interviewed in Scandinavia, she spoke great English.)

The risk of suicide or an attempt was highest in the first year of use. 'The vulnerable women are the youngest. That's where we saw the biggest effects and the negative effects. The women that took the pills for a long time were able to tolerate it better.' Of course, most pills were tested years ago on (perhaps larger-sized) American women in their twenties and thirties. 'But if you are a very young, very slim person, then you get a higher concentration in your blood of the pill's hormones,' said Dr Skovlund. Compared to the pills, users of the patch and the vaginal ring were even more at risk.[13] Shockingly, progestin-only hormonal implants quadrupled the increased risk of suicide, and although only around 4 per cent of women use the implant, the fact that it's impossible to remove at home if depression hits, unlike stopping the pill, is an added difficulty.

Dr Skovlund's latest research published in *The Lancet* looked at the effect of low and high dose hormonal coils on depression rates, and discovered that the Mirena coil with 52mg of the progestin levonorgestrel had a slightly higher risk of depression than the lower dose coils like the Kyleena with 19.5mg and the Jaydess, even better with 13.5mg of levonorgestrel. So the new, physically smaller, lower-dose coils might be a better option for younger women.[14]

Dr Skovlund believes people should take action and not suffer in silence. 'Women are very keen to put problems aside and live with a kind of low level of discomfort and say, "Oh, it's just me." And we've almost stopped ourselves complaining and asking for better contraception. We just think, "OK, we'll live with that." And that's what we're very much trying to change.'

WHEN YOU'RE FORCED TO LIVE WITH THE IMPLANT

Let's leave Denmark for a moment and go to North Devon in England to meet Jody Coyle, who is twenty-seven and had a horrendous experience on the progestin implant. Her contraceptive journey had always been rocky; it was clear from the off she was very sensitive to synthetic hormones. At fourteen years old she started taking the combined pill, which worked for a few months until a nurse realised at a check-up that Jody already suffered from migraines, and with that condition, the combined pill put her at higher risk of a stroke. Jody then went on to the progestin-only pill Cerazette instead. 'It gave me mood swings. Despite having no periods, my PMS symptoms got worse, and at fifteen I began to get anxiety too, but I stayed on it.' The Cerazette patient leaflet says common side effects which may affect up to 1 in 10 women include: 'mood altered, depressed mood, decreased sexual drive (libido).'[15]

When Jody was seventeen, she went to the Well Woman clinic at the GP and they put in the implant. 'I didn't know what to expect. I had constant bleeding, nine months straight.' She had numerous appointments, and asked for the implant to be taken out, to no avail. 'They kept telling me to wait a little bit longer and it would get better. It was really scary. I sometimes had thoughts of suicide.'

Jody was at college at the time, but found it hard to leave the house and struggled with low mood and anxiety. What made the difference for Jody was taking her mother with her to the next appointment, by which time she was eighteen. 'She advocated for me to get the implant out. It was really stressful.' There's a sense here that health professionals thought all that mattered was keeping young Jody on contraception; fear of teen pregnancy outweighed care for her mental health. 'They told me, "If you come off it, you'll get pregnant." I felt I didn't have any control over it.' After the implant had been removed, the clinic offered Jody the injection and the coil, but she refused and instead asked for an old-fashioned cervical cap (a barrier method which when used correctly with spermicide stops sperm getting into the uterus). Jody's cycle went back to normal, but she still battled with her mental health. At twenty-four, she was given medication when she was separately diagnosed with bipolar disorder.

However, since then, she has taken matters into her own hands. Now she's using condoms for sex, has been off medication for a year, watches out for mood dips before her periods, and feels in control. She has a job as a community development worker and a mental health advocate, as well as looking after her two children, aged five and seven. Thanks to her struggles with contraception, she was very aware of hormonal changes in her body after birth. She researched everything, and realised that she was suffering, as many women do, from vaginal atrophy when breastfeeding. She got help in the form of topical estrogen for the vulva, which is in such a tiny amount it does not affect mood. Now she runs an online community, the @HappyVulvaClub, helping other women experiencing the same issues.

Of course, the FSRH and sexual health clinics do suggest that if a pill or device doesn't suit someone and is affecting their mood, another one should be tried. 'It is important to acknowledge that some individuals report mood change during use of hormonal contraception whether the hormonal contraception is the cause of these changes or not.'[16] But how easy is it for younger women like Jody to advocate for themselves? Or to know the difference between their bodies and minds in a natural state, and with added synthetic hormones?

THE SWEDISH STUDY

British experts complained that the problem with Professor Lidegaard and Dr Skovlund's connection between hormonal contraception and mental health is that we can't prove causation; there could be other reasons for depression like genetics, family circumstances and environment. But Dr Therese Johansson of the Centre for Women's Mental Health During the Reproductive Lifespan at Uppsala University in Sweden had a great idea on how to eliminate some of those variables. She decided to do a contraceptive study of quarter of a million women from the UK Biobank — a giant medical database of patients — from birth to menopause. Crucially the Biobank has details of siblings, so Dr Johansson was also able to compare what happened over time to 7,000 pairs of sisters, with much the same genetics, in the same environment, when they used the combined pill, or not.

'I was looking through the scientific evidence available on mental health and the pill and the hormonal coil, and it was very different from what my own friends seemed to be experiencing,' she told me. 'I wanted to explain that difference.' Her 2023 study, published by Cambridge University Press,[17] gathered data on women's use of the pill and the time at which they were first diagnosed with depression or said they first experienced symptoms of depression. The UK results were similar to Professor Lidegaard's study of Danish women: the first two years of pill use were associated with a 79 per cent higher rate of depression compared to non-users. The risk got better after two years, but using the pill at all was associated with a slightly higher lifetime risk of depression.

But when Dr Johansson and her team looked at women in the Biobank who had also completed a mental health questionnaire, who were more likely to have experienced depressive symptoms, they found that teenagers starting the pill had a 130 per cent higher risk and adult starters had a 92 per cent raised risk. 'The powerful influence of contraceptive pills on teenagers can be ascribed to the hormonal changes already being caused by puberty, and to other life experiences,' said Dr Johansson. The pill might be pushing girls already at risk of depression to tipping point. And there's more: Dr Johannsson's next investigation will be on other forms of hormonal contraception.

Following up on these studies, a 2023 discussion paper on The Oral Contraceptive Pill and Adolescents' Mental Health[18] looked at Danish doctors' appointments for antidepressants in the year after teenagers started the contraceptive pill. The line on the antidepressant-use graph rises steadily over the months from starting birth control. The analysis shows 'a very clear break in teenage girls' mental health trajectories: soon after initiating oral contraception, there is an increase in the likelihood of psychiatric contact, of a depression diagnosis, and of antidepressant use'. The academics eliminated girls with previous at-risk behaviours or mental health problems and found that 15 per cent of the 65 per cent upsurge in teen antidepressant use seemed directly connected to first-time pill use. Doctors who were most likely to prescribe the pill to the youngest patients also had higher levels of return for antidepressants. They said: 'Being assigned to a high-prescribing physician strongly predicts pill use by age sixteen and leads to worse mental health outcomes between ages sixteen to eighteen.'

THE WHOLE TRUTH AND NOTHING BUT THE TRUTH?

There has been quite a lot of work done over the years on the link between depression and the different forms of contraception, but some of this research seems to have been left languishing in the bottom drawer or mis-reported. Here's something I've learned writing books on the menopause and the pill: never trust the title or the press release summary of a science paper. A 2021 study in *BJOG*, the official academic research journal of the Royal College of Obstetricians and Gynaecologists, was headlined: 'There is no association between combined oral hormonal contraceptives and depression: a Swedish register-based cohort study'.[19] Researchers looked at a database of over 700,000 women aged fifteen to twenty-five with no prior antidepressant treatment or psychiatric diagnoses. That all sounded pretty reliable, but then I read the results in detail and discovered that every single hormonal contraceptive method — *except* the combined pill — caused an increased risk of depression. For the progestin pill there was a 13 per cent extra risk, the implant 38 per cent, patch or ring 43 per cent, and IUD 59 per cent. So, all the progestin-based methods had an increased risk of depression. Why did the journal headline pick out the one method that (weirdly) bucked the worrying trend? How do they get away with skewing the results in reputable medical journals?

It's hard not to get paranoid reporting this story. Here's another biased headline: 'A first-choice combined oral contraceptive influences general well-being in healthy women',[20] from the journal *Fertility and Sterility*. Sounds super. But read closer and you find that the contraceptive pill *negatively* affected well-being. Indeed, the conclusion (but not the headline) refers to a 'statistically significant reduction' in well-being. This was a 'gold standard' double-blind (i.e. no one, not even the scientists, knew who was on a pill or a placebo) randomised controlled trial in 2017 in Sweden. The doctors gave 340 women aged eighteen to thirty-five a combined levonorgestrel progestin and synthetic estrogen pill (similar to Microgynon or Rigevidon) or a placebo for three months, with monthly breaks for bleeds. Well-being went down by over 4 per cent in the pill group and self-reported positive thoughts, self-control and vitality also fell. 'We found no statistically significant effects on depressive symptoms,' said the summary. But obviously the sort of self-selecting adult woman who willingly enters a contraceptive trial will be very different from a teenage girl, and the study stopped after three months. Even so, the immediate lowering of mood is interesting. Serious depression can be recorded from prescriptions or requests for therapy, but feeling a bit down or 'meh' is just something women put up with, and it mostly goes unrecorded.

The worship of the randomised controlled trial (RCT)

above all else sometimes seems obsessive. In the *British Journal of Psychiatry Open* in 2021, academics looked at more than three thousand studies on the subject of hormonal contraception and depressive symptoms and concluded that only twelve randomised controlled trials were relevant.[21] From those chosen trials, they concluded that 'hormonal contraceptive use does not lead to an increase in depressive symptoms in adult women. Future studies should include first-time users, to confirm the results in young women.' But the number of women in that total of twelve trials was 5,833. Tiny. Almost as small as our diverse poll of 4,000 women for the *Pill Revolution*, which showed the opposite result with depression and anxiety affecting over a third of respondents. I know polls are not an exact science, but the millions in the big database surveys did have actual diagnoses of depression, and those were totally ignored here. And look at the bias in the last quote – these results must be 'confirmed' in young women, not questioned. It's as though there's a conspiracy to make the complainers quietly disappear.

MANY WOMEN ARE QUIETLY HAVING A PILL MELTDOWN

When I said I was writing this book, dozens of women who have taken the combined pill contacted me through my @pillscandal Instagram to tell me how it negatively affected their mental health. Some had been on antidepressants to counteract the depressive action of the pill, and hadn't joined up the dots until they had stopped using birth control. Some never reported the mental health problems to their doctor, blaming themselves until they stopped the pill and perked up. There were short, sharp messages like this: 'I was on Dianette in my later teens. It made me so mentally unwell I nearly walked in front of a bus. It also exacerbated my already horrendous PMDD [premenstrual dysphoric disorder] and made my migraines worse. Clear skin though' (@Ms.soundbird). (I've previously mentioned the warning on the rare risk of psychiatratric disorders in the Dianette patient leaflet on page 60.)

Of course, not everyone needs to a have a tendency to depression or PMDD to be suddenly floored by the pill. When Abby Fry was twenty-two, happily studying Marketing and Management at the University of East Anglia, she went on Rigevidon (the NHS's cheapest ethinylestradiol and levonorgestrel combined pill), partly because she was experiencing adult acne. 'I was in second year at university, and it did help my skin a little bit, but then made it worse. I started getting side effects of low mood. I was snappy and had really high anxiety. I had no problem with my coursework before, but I suddenly struggled to do it at all.' Eventually Abby had a full-blown meltdown. 'I'd never felt so low before.' Her mother, Paula Fry, a City executive who opened up about her own fluctuating hormones in our second menopause documentary, advised Abby to stop taking the pill.

Within a week she started feeling better. 'I realised I'd been horrible to my friends; I'd been a cow. I'd even been going to drop out of university.' She remained petrified of the pill, but she also didn't want to have acne again, so she tried Yasmin (ethinylestradiol and drospirenone) for a few months, but it did not make much difference, so she dropped it. She is looking for a new solution for her skin, perhaps the drug spironolactone, which has shown good results over six months in lowering acne for some women in a 2023 study.[22] Abby is now twenty-seven and works in London as a fashion brand manager. 'I was under a black cloud for a year at university. I can't believe I nearly gave up something I loved for the pill.'

A PILL FOR BARBIE?

It's interesting that Abby considered Yasmin for her skin because it has a popular reputation as a 'feminising' pill, with its anti-androgenic progestin drospirenone, which is derived from spironolactone, the diuretic which also some-times works as an anti-acne drug. Along with clear skin, some patients also found the synthetic estrogen in Yasmin made their breasts bigger, while the diuretic helped slim away any bloating. In many ways, it was a teenage girl's dream drug, the pill Barbie might choose.

The combined drospirenone and ethinylestradiol pill is known as Yasmin and Yaz (which is now discontinued in the UK but still available as the generic pill Eloine). Yaz has a lower dose of estrogen and a four-day bleed break, and Yasmin has slightly more estrogen and a seven-day break. In America, pharmaceutical companies can advertise on television, newspapers and social media, and Yaz was sold not just as contraception, but as the first 'lifestyle pill' that would help with mental health. The manufacturers Bayer put out a 2008 advert which showed a young blonde woman in a yellow vest punching away the giant words 'Fatigue', 'Bloating', 'Moodiness' and 'Acne', and the headline read: 'Ready for birth control that goes beyond?' Yaz was described as 'the first and only contraceptive proven to treat physical and emotional pre-menstrual symptoms severe enough to affect your life, a condition doctors call PMDD'. Those treatable symptoms could also include 'feeling anxious', 'increased appetite' and 'irritability'. By 2009, Yaz was celebrated in women's magazines and became the best-selling oral contraceptive on the American market, making $700,000 million a year.

You'll not be surprised to hear Yaz didn't do exactly what it said on the tin. The Food and Drug Administration (FDA) said Bayer had exaggerated the mental health and other benefits of the pill and failed to make clear the risks. Bayer was punished and told to finance a $20 million corrective television and magazine campaign giving the full version of the truth. The risks were serious. While the newer drospirenone progestin worked for some women, it had disastrous effects on others, particularly in terms of an increased risk for blood clots, even in younger women. The FDA put out a warning about drospirenone in 2012,[23] which was in Yaz, Yasmin and a number of other pills. In July 2012, Bayer notified its stockholders that there were more than 12,000 lawsuits pending against the company and they had already settled 1,977 cases for $402.6 million, around $212,000 per case.[24] Soon there were 19,000 cases. I'll cover the blood clot risks on Yaz and Yazmin in more detail in Chapter 8. The Consumer Law Group in

Canada started a class action lawsuit around clots and deep vein thrombosis (DVT), but the women's complaints also included severe anxiety and depression.[25]

It's hard to prove legally that depression or anxiety is the result of taking a contraceptive pill, whereas a blood clot in a previously healthy teenager is suspicious. But her own experience and the anecdotal stories of thousands of women using Yaz and Yasmin led British journalist Holly Grigg-Spall to write the 2013 book *Sweetening The Pill: Or how we got hooked on hormonal birth control.*[26] Holly had initially been pleased with the skin-clearing, breast-enhancing, weight-loss effects of Yasmin, but after two years that began to change. 'I had been feeling depressed for some time. I felt my confidence and energy were evaporating. I had little motivation and struggled to think clearly. Bouts of anxiety and paranoia had me at home alone calling my boyfriend twice an hour to check he wasn't dead and caused me to leave parties convinced I had burned all my bridges with my friends. Nor did I mention the constant sense of dread that convinced me some terrible event was just around the corner.'[27]

Holly found her experience reflected by friends on Yasmin and on online chatrooms like the Yaz Survivors' Forum, people feeling that they had experienced a complete change in personality. She began investigating further and wrote a magazine article. She came off Yasmin, but soon after went on another brand of pill. Eventually, she came off the pill for a few months: 'I felt lighter,' she wrote. 'A rush of positive emotions let me feel happiness, excitement and enthusiasm.'[28] And then, worried about pregnancy and not in the best of mental health, she changed her mind about starting the pill again: 'Like a victim of Stockholm Syndrome, I went back to taking it.'

It was only when she moved to America with her boyfriend in 2009 that Holly finally kicked what was, in many ways, an addiction. She read the book *The Pill: Are You Sure It's for You?* by Jane Bennett and Alexandra Pope, and realised that the synthetic hormones were changing her psychological state. On a recent podcast, Holly said: 'There wasn't Instagram, there wasn't people sharing information the way they are on TikTok . . . There was an underground network of people finding each other. Most of the people I spoke to felt very isolated and didn't think it happened to anybody else. Most of them blamed themselves.'[29] Holly wrote a number of blogs, a book, and became a producer on the 2022 independent American documentary, *The Business of Birth Control* along with actor Rikki Lake and filmmaker Abby Epstein.[30] The film looked at the feminist movement, the pill's racist legacy, and talked to parents whose children had died on the pill, as well as looking for alternatives to hormonal birth control. Holly went on to lead an online workshop helping women to come off hormonal birth control.[31]

COMING OFF THE PILL

The sense that Holly felt addicted to the pill makes sense, when you think about the long-term good and bad effects of synthetic hormones. We've looked at the effects of starting the pill, but what about coming off it? There are short-term side effects like irregular periods and perhaps a return of acne or the infamous 'mood swings', but most women seem to cope. But what if your liver and body is detoxing after years or decades on synthetic hormones, and what if your body came to rely on those synthetic hormones as their own? Asha Knight is a television distribution manager in London, and she contacted me to tell me how coming off the combined pill after seventeen years crashed her whole life, leaving her with unbearable insomnia, anxiety and auditory hallucinations. It was so bad she was eventually referred by her GP to The Priory, a mental health and rehabilitation clinic in London.

So many of these stories seem to begin with teenage acne, which is why Asha started the combined pill Dianette at thirteen or fourteen years old. That was mostly fine until she went to university and changed to Microgynon (which has a slightly lower dose of synthetic estrogen and progestin, different from Dianette). 'I was instantly low. Then I changed to Yasmin, and it was a wonder-pill for me from twenty-one to thirty,' said Asha. 'Then when I stopped taking Yasmin to try for a baby, I just totally lost my marbles.' Being pill-free was a nightmare for her. She had no previous mental health issues, but within a month of coming off Yasmin, she developed 'massive anxiety over things that never used to rattle me, and a weird kind of insomnia – it wasn't that my mind was racing, but I'd put my head on the pillow, fall asleep, and be jolted awake twenty seconds later.'

Asha said of her husband: 'Imagine his surprise after he married me – "Where is my wife?" It was a complete shock to both of us. I was on the pill for so long that whatever version of myself it created became reality.' Before starting treatment at The Priory, she was prescribed the sleeping pill zopiclone and antidepressants. Her symptoms were worst in the first half of her monthly cycle when natural progesterone is low. The insomnia was diagnosed as a severe case of hypnic jerks, those twitches you make as you fall asleep. Her anxiety was so bad that it led to auditory hallucinations, but she was always aware they weren't real. 'One night I thought I was batshit crazy. I heard the voice of Morgan Freeman (it was definitely him) and he told me to try harder.' Asha laughed, but it can't have been funny at the time. She was signed off work for months and spent six weeks as a day-patient at the Priory, going home to try to sleep at her parents' house every night and gradually weaning off zopiclone. She eventually got good one-to-one psychotherapy and worked out some coping techniques, although the insomnia didn't fully go away. That is, until Asha became pregnant. 'Progesterone is nature's Valium and I felt happy being pregnant on all that progesterone.' It is likely that she naturally had low or erratic progesterone, which the Dianette and Yasmin had topped up. 'Maybe I went on the pill so young my body and mind never had a chance to adapt to a natural hormonal cycle, never regulated itself,' said Asha.

Asha had her first baby, a boy, and it wasn't easy, as she suffered from post-natal anxiety and the insomnia returned. She also coped with two miscarriages, which she believes might be to do with progesterone deficiency. Then she had a little girl, and the crash afterwards came again. While the coping mechanisms for the insomnia helped, it became so debilitating that she decided to try the progestin-only pill. 'The insomnia disappeared, quite literally, overnight.' She is sleeping at a last and is looking into a body-identical progesterone too. You wonder why none of the medical and psychiatric professionals considered a progesterone deficiency. Asha wants more people to know about the mental health risks of coming on and off the pill. 'It's about how you absorb the hormones. I'm not saying don't go on the pill, but be knowledgeable and informed about it.'

Conversely, some women who may have slight progesterone deficiency or are sensitive to hormonal fluctuations find the progestin-only pill really helps steady mental health. Maya Oppenheim, the women's correspondent at *The Independent* who tells her abortion story in Chapter 11, told me: 'I found the pill really useful for PMS; it massively alleviated it.' She was on a progestin-only pill (desogestrel) throughout her twenties and said: 'It levelled out any peaks and troughs.' Before she was eighteen, she was on the combined pill Microgynon (ethinylestradiol and levonorgestrel), which had a bad psychological effect on her. Changing to progestin-only 'made me feel so much better'. Maya's experience makes me think we should be assertive consumers, not submissive patients, when it comes to choosing the right pill. Just as we'd return a dress that didn't fit to ASOS or Zara, so we should send back the pill until we find one that fits properly.

A WINDOW INTO THE BRAIN

For so long, women's worries about brain changes on the pill have been dismissed; we have been disbelieved by some medical professionals about our suffering. It's very weird that some academics insist on keeping the epidemiology and neuroscience around hormonal contraception and depression in separate silos, while making sure the door is guarded by a rigorous adherence to the randomised controlled trial. If you work in this space, and you've spoken to another sensible, articulate working woman who has burst into tears remembering her mental hell on contraception, you want to scream at the institutional fatberg of resistance to the truth of lived experience. This institutional denial, the downplaying of complications by major contraceptive providers, is doing women a gross disservice.

What's going on here? Is it a sort of academic paternalism restricting our freedom to complain, or believe in our complaints, because it is in society's interest for women to keep calm and carry on taking the pill? Is it a paranoia about teen pregnancy? The evidence on synthetic hormones' risky effect on the brain, particularly the teenage brain, is overwhelming.

Increasingly, psychiatrists are asking women the simple question: 'Are you on the pill?' Professor Kulkarni is the director of the Psychiatric Research Centre at Monash University, Australia, and from a practising and academic point of view, tells it as she sees it. 'Currently, all oral contraceptive pills may cause mood changes . . . Hormonal contraception is known to precipitate or perpetuate depression in some patients. The link between oral contraceptive pills and depression relates to the amount and type of progestogen [progestin] contained in these pills.'[32] She also noted that many of the older combined pills, which contain ethinylestradiol, are linked to severe mood problems, and that newer pills containing plant-based, body-identical estrogen may be better tolerated.

But as neuroscience and brain imaging technology advances, we now have proof before our eyes of the effect of synthetic versus natural hormones. My final Scandi scientist is Søren Vinther Larsen, a neurobiologist at the Rigshospitalet in Copenhagen, who also worked with Dr Johansson on the UK Biobank study. Dr Larsen scanned the brains of fifty-three women, sixteen of whom were on the pill, mostly the combined one. The PET (positron emission tomography) scan uses a mildly radioactive drug to show up areas of your brain where cells are more active than normal, and he wanted to see what happened to the serotonin receptors when a woman was on hormonal contraception. Serotonin is a hormone and neurotransmitter, sometimes known as 'the happy chemical', which plays a major role in regulating mood. Low levels of serotonin in the brain are associated with depression. Serotonin is also involved in appetite and digestion, bone health, sex and sleep. In other words, you want some.

'We found that healthy adult women who used oral contraceptives had around 10 per cent lower global brain serotonin 4 receptor binding compared to non-users,' said Dr Larsen. It looks like the synthetic hormones were partially blocking serotonin. 'This is only baby steps. This is a small study, so it's giving us an idea. I want to do a full randomised controlled trial, but so far, we think this could show a plausible link between oral contraceptive use and an increased risk of depressive episodes.' A longitudinal study, following women over years, will be finished in summer 2024.

The largest brain change, around 13 per cent, was in the hippocampus, which regulates memory and emotion. 'It could be that the small change caused by oral contraceptives could be a tipping point for some women. It's important to note that none of the women in our study were already depressed,' said Dr Larsen. Even if you find Dr Larsen's paper tricky to read, it's worth scrolling down just to look at the brain scans. Women on oral contraception show paler colours in the brain; the throbbing patch of red action is dimmed.[33] The research has also raised the question about whether the pill interferes with antidepressants like SSRIs (selective serotonin reuptake inhibitors), which are thought to work by increasing serotonin levels in the brain. Dr Larsen is also interested to discover the effect of the pill on teenage brains. 'I would really love to look into that because that's maybe one of the reasons why we see higher risk in the young ones. But due to using radioactivity in the scans, we don't have these young ones. We can only have them from eighteen years old.'

SOME HORMONAL HOPE

While most teens are too young to benefit from Dr Larsen's trials, Millennials and Gen Z are having plenty of conversations on TikTok and Instagram and developing their own information networks that circumvent official-dom. Younger women are discussing the effects of different pills on mental health, getting information from apps like Clue, and reviewing products on sites like The Lowdown. There's a lot of interest in body-identical estrogens, a copy of women's own hormones, derived from yams or soy. Dr Annabel Sowemimo, who works in sexual and reproductive health in Leicester, says she has found that pills like Qlaira, which contains the body-identical estradiol plus progestin, are 'worth trying for women who have really struggled with their mood on the other pills, but we need more research'. Pills with body-identical estrogen include Qlaira, Zoely and Drovelis in the UK and Naemis and Nextstellis in the US. But guess what? The body-identical pills are more expensive in the US, and in the UK they are not offered in most NHS areas because of higher costs.

In Australia, Professor Kulkarni and her team completed a pilot trial in 2021 on the mental health effects of Zoely,[34] a combined pill which contains the progestin NOMAC (nomegestrol acetate) and body-identical estrogen, (17-beta estradiol). They recruited forty-nine women who attended the Alfred women's mental health clinic and had been diagnosed with PMDD. The majority also had a history of trauma. Almost 75 per cent of patients reported a subjective positive mood response and reduced depression, anxiety and stress, and 63 per cent stayed on the medication. Around 20 per cent of women reported side effects as the main reason for discontinuing. The researchers said women who develop depression early after taking other oral contraceptive pills may tolerate Zoely better, and the progestin NOMAC has a good safety profile for clots, too. As usual, we need someone somewhere to pay for a larger randomised controlled trial, but it's exciting to know that better-tolerated body-identical pills like Zoely are in the works, not just for women with previous mood disorders.

SPEAK TRUTH TO POWER — AND YOUR DOCTOR

What have we learned from this evisceration of the pill and mental health? That we need to speak truth to power, that women need to advocate for themselves, log any changes when they start a pill on an app or their phone, and be ready to ask their doctor for a different form of contraception. Otherwise, years and lives can be wasted. And if it was hard for the women in this chapter like Kirsty and Jody to be heard by their doctors, how much worse is it for those whose main language is not English, or people living with disabilities? As the contraceptive pill becomes increasingly available over the counter in pharmacies in America and the UK, who will track the mental health outcomes of those women, except the women themselves? There's a massive responsibility for the medical establishment to open a wider, more honest conversation around hormonal contraception and mental health.

Now women know the truth, they won't keep calm and carry on.

CHAPTER FOUR

SEX

The contraceptive pill has not merely brought women workplace and educational mobility – it has also brought sexual mobility. Literally. The joy of sex without fear of pregnancy means we can indulge in spontaneous combustion whenever and wherever we like: on trains, planes and automobiles; on kitchen counters, on the stairs, on the roof; in parks on warm summer nights; on the beach and in the sea; in offices, libraries and broom cupboards; in the woods; in nature. Without the barrier of condoms, the pill generation roamed wild – without leaving any seeds.

HOW DOES THE PILL AFFECT YOUR LIBIDO?

This glorious unleashing of pleasure and opportunity began in the Swinging Sixties and Shagadelic Seventies and continues into the TikTok Twenties. And yet – and I'm sorry to bring you back down to earth from the mile-high club with a bump here – in our 4,000-women *Pill*

Revolution survey, 21 per cent of pill-users interviewed said their sex drive had become lower. Many people don't particularly notice the change at the time; only afterwards, when they come off the pill.

Now that more women know there is no need to have a fake bleed on the pill, it has probably increased sexual activity worldwide — a 2023 survey by the cycle app Flo found that almost half of British women avoided having sex on their periods,[1] so that freedom is a bonus, and even fans of the occasional bleed will take packets back-to-back on holiday. But the pill also made some of us feel much less sexy, particularly in the longer term.

That happened to me after spending most of my student life at the University of Glasgow on Microgynon. It was only when I stopped that combined pill and changed to the diaphragm that I realised there was this mad, mid-month craving that needed to be satisfied around ovulation, and that I was just that bit keener on any available activity once I was released from synthetic hormones.

But many people on the pill experience a much more serious loss of libido, and it can make them absolutely miserable and destroy relationships. Passion flatlines for them. Sometimes penetrative sex becomes a Victorian-style 'Lie back and think of England!' chore to maintain a partnership and please a man (or indeed any person with a penis) and not ourselves. I was thinking about the one-fifth of women who say their desire has changed on the pill, and before I dug into the science, I wanted to know more about how they felt, so I posted this question on my @pillscandal and @menoscandal Instagram: 'Feeling hot . . . or not?

Did your libido change when taking the contraceptive pill?' and explained I was writing a book. The comments poured in immediately, and lots agreed to go public.

'Just spotted your latest post and let out an audible "Ha!" What libido? I'm thirty-three, fit and healthy, with no children and a husband I'm luckily still very much attracted to. But libido is non-existent. I changed over from Microgynon to the mini-pill (they're constantly changing my brand) and although my weight has slightly changed, my lack of sex drive is the thing I've noticed most . . . I've spoken to friends who've come off the pill and they've advised it was "life changing".' @sexualbeanbag

'Yes! Was like someone turned my libido light off when I went on the pill. Came off it for that reason in my twenties.' @Deborellahollywood

'Not hot – actually I became freezing – libido died a death therefore rendering the contraceptive pill a pointless medication, as I believe you actually have to have sex to get pregnant.' @Traynor_swift

'Not libido but my natural lubrication reduced, hence I used KY and Durex lubes which caused recurrent infections because of the irritating ingredients which in turn led to vaginismus [clenching of the vaginal muscles] which affected my libido! It also made me depressed, which affected my libido too.' @Samtalkssex

'God, we get so trained into gaslighting ourselves – let's be honest, our doctors would never have even considered this a thing and still don't. I'm being told to use lube by my female doctor when I told her I have no sexual desire and this is not normal.' @minky_67

'I found at times the idea of sex was a foreign abstract concept which just seemed like a strange and kind gross thing to do! My body craved sex again when I came off it.' @lo_is_af

'OMG yes. This was the nineties in Canada. I told my doctor that it positively extinguished any thoughts of sex except for a tiny, wavering, ephemeral little flicker just before my period.' @trueirv

And so it continued for pages (of course, my followers are a biased sample.) There was only one positive response:

'No, it made me feel liberated lol.' @Cathyrhi2

THE LOWDOWN ON LOST DESIRE

There's an unacknowledged protest group out there, and lowered sex drive affects women on both the combined and progestin-only pill, as well as the implant, injection and ring. No one in that small sample above complained about the hormonal coil. On The Lowdown contraceptive review site, reports of lost desire were even more prevalent, but the moderators do point out that people are often more likely to file a review if they have a complaint about a particular form of contraception. When it's all fabulous, pill-users are probably off and away having sex. Anyway, The Lowdown results were that 51 per cent had lowered libido on the progestin-only pill, 48 per cent on the combined pill, 50 per on the patch and implant, 54 per cent on the vaginal ring and 56 per cent on the injection. Interestingly, on the hormonal coil, 47 per had no change of sex drive and only 29 per cent said they had a drop in libido.

So, anecdotally, the coil may be a sexier option for some women, possibly because the hormones are differently absorbed or because some women start ovulating again after a while on the coil and therefore stay perky. But whether it's 50 per cent or just 10 per cent of pill-users struggling to find more joy in sex, the number doesn't really matter. It's the fact this conversation about libido isn't being had enough in public, and that women, trans men and non-binary people – and their relationships – are genuinely suffering.

Let's find out what the professionals think about our crashing sex drives. Under 'loss of libido' the NHS suggests maybe changing your pill, and that's it – a very short entry, with no explanation of precisely why this is happening. Planned Parenthood also advises that 'women with decreased sexual desire may want to try a different birth control pill' and there's a serious article on female Hypoactive Sexual Desire Disorder (HSDD), a big medical term for the bio-psycho-social effects that can lower libido, including stress, anxiety, trauma, difficult relationships, body image issues, and use of antidepressants or other drugs. Previously HSDD was more unpleasantly labelled by the Victorians as 'frigidity'. But hormonal contraception is still not seen as a major culprit on the libido front.

In the UK, the textbook *Contraception: Your Questions Answered* by Professor John Guillebaud and Dr Anne MacGregor gives the matter of libido very short shrift.[2] 'Again, encourage women to continue with the method for at least three months. If symptoms persist consider changing the POP to a different progestogen or consider a different method.' The other major guidebook *Contraception Made Easy*, by Dr Laura Percy and Dr Diana Mansour,[3] makes a few mentions of libido when discussing different products, but it emphasises again and again that 'no causal association has been found'[4] between hormonal contraception and lowered sex drive. It adds on the low-dose combined pill: 'There is no clear evidence of an association between use of combined hormonal contraceptives containing 20 micrograms or less of ethinylestradiol and libido.'[5]

To the contrary: there is a truckload of scientific evidence out there connecting hormonal contraception and lowered sexual desire. Just pop 'libido' and 'pill' into the search engine of *The Journal of Sexual Medicine* for a deluge of studies. So, why are trainee doctors not being properly alerted to women's struggles with libido and hormonal contraception? Why doesn't this merit at least a page or even a paragraph in medical textbooks? Why is it hushed up? Is it because contraception is still seen as only about the repression of pregnancy, and not the expression of desire? And let's just fact-check that assertion above, that lower dose combined pills have no effect on libido. In a 2013 study,[6] women using combined pills with the smallest dose of estrogen available (15 micrograms), reported decreased libido, while the majority of people using pills with higher doses of estrogen reported no change, or less often, an increase or a decrease in libido.

THE EFFECT ON DESIRE AND AROUSAL

Libido is a complex creature, affected by the daily weather of hormones, arguments, stress, exhaustion, past trauma, present boredom and the waxing or waning attraction to a specific person or a fantasy in masturbation. But there are genuine physical changes that affect libido, and teasing those out from other feelings may help us understand whether hormonal contraception is affecting us or not. As you might expect by now, the Nordic countries are on the case, and another Scandi scientist has done some interesting research into the combined pill and libido. Niklaus Zethraeus, an associate professor at the Karolinska Institute in Stockholm, and his team recruited 340 women who were randomised to a combined pill (levonorgestrel and ethinylestradiol) or a placebo (dummy pill) over three months, and asked them how they felt. The researchers used a set of statements called the Profile of Female Sexual Function (PFSF) that recognise some of the complexities. They include:

'I felt like having sex'
'I was unhappy about my lack of interest in sex'

'Getting aroused took for ever'
'I felt sexually numb'
'I felt disappointed by my lack of interest in sex'
'I lacked sexual desire'
'I reached orgasm easily'

The researchers found that people in the pill group were significantly more likely to report decreased sexual desire, arousal and pleasure compared to non-users. So, the process of fancying and foreplay was trickier, but eventual responsiveness remained the same and orgasms were normal.[7]

While libido is seen to fall in some randomised controlled trials, others show no change. Experts think that could be to do with the different types of progestin in different brands of pills – and each woman's individual reaction to it. In some studies, nomegestrol acetate, drospirenone (found on its own and in pills like Yasmin) and dienogest have reported a positive effect on sexual response,[8] whereas the more androgenic progestins like levonorgestrel and norgestrel seem more likely to have a negative effect. But there's no way to guess how you will react: we remain guinea pigs using trial and error until better information – and better contraception – is provided.

The hormonal coil was found to cause no alteration in sexual functioning in several studies, and in a study of 200 women,[9] some even found that their desire and arousal improved on the coil. There's a good 2019 summary of all this, 'The Potential of Hormonal Contraception to

Influence Female Sexuality',[10] which looks at eighty different pieces of research in the area and concludes: 'This review suggests that hormonal contraception can cause female sexual response impairment . . . Several studies have linked hormonal contraception to negative effects of sexual function, but also to a neutral effect, or an improvement in the sexual domains, compared to women who do not use hormonal methods.' The authors' final suggestion? 'There are so many factors that affect the sexual response, it seems appropriate to incorporate women's sexual health into contraceptive counselling and to maintain the assessment of sexual function as an integral part of follow-up consultations.' A brilliant plan.

THE 'OBJECTIONABLE INJECTABLE'

As we have seen, women report different levels of libido on different contraception, and it looks like the Depo-Provera injection comes out bottom of the league table. Aside from the anecdotal evidence on The Lowdown, an American study of almost 2,000 women[11] on different forms of contraception found that the injection – which contains a large dose of the progestin medroxyprogesterone acetate – caused 37 per cent of women to 'lose interest in sex' after six months of use. That compared to a loss of interest of 18 per cent for women on the non-hormonal copper coil. Looking at that research, I noticed 80 per cent of the Depo users were Black and 20 per cent white; for decades there has been a campaign against the racial and ethnic disparities in use of the drug, the overpromotion of the injection in certain communities, and the disproportionate use of it on women who have learning disabilities.[12] Indeed, in the seventies, the Women's Liberation Movement ran a campaign against Depo, calling it the 'objectionable injectable'. Aside from plummeting libido, it also has some of the worst reported side effects, including lowered bone density, which increases risk of fractures,[13] and when the medroxyprogesterone acetate progestin in Depo is used in menopausal hormone replacement therapy, it has a small increased risk of breast cancer.[14] The Depo injection may be convenient, but the downsides are serious.

@Traynor_swift, who we heard from above about libido disappearing on the pill, had an even more appalling time on Depo-Provera, which gave her panic attacks and weight gain. 'The pill left me emotionally flat and joyless . . . and Depo-Provera even worse. I believe it's been used on male sex offenders,' she added. I shot down that internet rabbit hole straightaway, and I can confirm that, according to the Houston Law Review, in 1986 Texas courts granted sex offenders probation instead of continued imprisonment if they agreed to regular Depo-Provera injections.[15] 'When combined with psychological treatment of the deviant behaviour, Depo-Provera reduces offensive behaviour related to sexual fantasies and performance in 70 to 80 per cent of men under treatment.' Obviously female hormones act differently on men, but it's certainly off-putting.

HOW HORMONAL CHEMISTRY AFFECTS OUR SEXUAL CHEMISTRY

The reporting of levels of libido by women cannot help but be subjective, both from the point of view of the woman and the researcher. But to explain what's happening – and it's clear that something *is* happening to large numbers of women out there in bedrooms – we can just look at the mechanics of the body on contraception. Natural estrogen, which makes women feel sexy, is usually produced much less because users of the combined pill are being fed a low dose of synthetic estrogen. The steady, often high doses of synthetic progestins thicken cervical mucus to block sperm and prevent ovulation, so cyclical desire also lessens.

The other massive effect, which has been known for years, is that most progestin contraception lowers female 'free' testosterone, which helps fuel libido, by increasing the amount of sex hormone binding globulin (SHBG) in the body. Think of SHBG as a sort of hormonal super-glue that takes your horniness right out of circulation. And here's the double whammy: since both estrogen and testosterone receptors all over the vagina contribute to lubrication, having low testosterone can cause dryness, pain and increase the likelihood of urinary tract infections.

Temporary loss of testosterone levels is bad enough, but way back in 2006, researchers measured sex hormone binding globulin (SHBG) in pill-users and non-users.[16] Women on the pill had higher SHBG, but they discovered that this effect continued after stopping. Low testosterone might lead to continuing sexual, metabolic and mental health consequences. Three months afterwards, the women's SHBG levels were still four times higher than non-users of the pill. The testosterone was still chained up. This explained day-to-day observations by those doctors over the previous seven years that women still suffered lowered libido long after stopping the pill. (Although happily our Instagram sample seems to show people eventually getting their mojo back.)

Dr Claudia Panzer, the Colorado endocrinologist who led the small study of 124 women said then: 'The use of oral contraceptives led to changes in the synthesis of SHBG which were not completely reversible in our time frame of observation. This can lead to lower levels of "unbound" [free] testosterone, which is thought to play a major role in female sexual health. It would be important to conduct long-term studies to see if these increased SHBG changes are permanent . . . It is important for physicians prescribing oral contraceptives to point out to their patients' potential sexual side effects, such as decreased desire, arousal, decreased lubrication and increased sexual pain. Also, if women present with these complaints, it is crucial to recognize the link between sexual dysfunction and the oral contraceptive and not to attribute these complaints solely to psychological causes.'[17]

Although it is scientifically proven that many progestins affect our testosterone levels, we're not told this upfront by GPs, and sometimes years and even decades go by without us realising. (It's not even the fault of GPs, many of whom were trained long ago with the outdated binary idea that estrogen was a female hormone and testosterone was solely male.) But that lack of knowledge is very upsetting for women who realise in hindsight that they have suffered unnecessarily. Here are a couple more Instagram comments:

'I came off the pill six months ago. I didn't realise how foggy it's made me. My periods are now normal, no mood swings around my period and my libido is normal. So sad I spent years on it to be honest. My own daughter will not be doing the same!' @sophy.green.x

'I was on the pill constantly from 1992 to 2013. I experienced all the indicators of chemical castration but didn't realise that's what it was at the time. Zero libido, depression, fatigue, weight gain. It destroyed my relationship with my partner. I didn't even try having children, that's how bad it got. I came off the pill at 40 but by then it was too late. My libido came back, but my partner and I had split up, and it's difficult to conceive in your forties, plus not many men want to start a family that late. I'm 50 now and never had children. The pill stole my life.' @universal_unfolding

Aside from the effect of hormonal contraception on desire in our brains, it can also have an uncomfortable direct effect on our bodies, particularly around the vulva. You've probably heard of the microbiome in the stomach, but it might come as a surprise that there is also a vaginal microbiome or 'vaginome' (which sounds like a cartoon gnome) that is full of the good bacteria Lactobacillus and it needs to stay healthy to keep your vagina lubricated, the skin of your vulva plump and healthy, and to prevent urinary tract infections. The delicate pH balance of microbes in the vaginal microbiome can be altered by synthetic hormones (and spermicides)[18] that can cause negative effects like bacterial vaginosis (BV), a discharge that often smells slightly fishy. Estrogen supports Lactobacillus growth, but if the pill lowers your natural estrogen levels, you may get atrophy, where the tissue of the vulva and vagina gets dry and papery. This can cause itching and even bleeding, and makes it easier to get infections like thrush (candida). Women who use contraceptives containing synthetic estrogen also seem more likely to get oral or vaginal candida infections.[19]

Combined contraceptives sometimes encourage a stable microbiome, but many progestin-only pills have shown an increase in problems like vaginal atrophy. A 2023 study in the *Journal of Sexual Medicine*,[20] which involved examining the arousal of 130 pill-users and non-users watching 'sexual films', found that women who used pills containing androgenic progestins 'experienced decreased vaginal blood flow and lubrication as well as higher rates of self-reported vaginal bleeding and female sexual arousal disorder'. Over on The Lowdown review site, the vaginal dryness ratings (possibly from very irritated users) for different methods came out with the vaginal ring and patch performing worst with 42 per cent having problems, the combined pill at 41 per cent, the progestin-only pill and implant at 39 per cent, and the hormonal coil doing best at 23 per cent.[21] Women who experience dryness or urinary tract infections may want to top up with a long-term prescription from their GP of local vaginal estrogen gel or an estrogen pessary, which aids collagen and elasticity, as well as helping the microbiome to function better. (Lube might help during sex, but it has no permanent effect on improving dryness or estrogen levels.) Probiotics may also help the vaginal microbiome. When it goes wrong, it can seriously affect you, your libido and your whole sex life.

WHAT'S VULVODYNIA?

Suzie Bishop described herself to me as an 'average 34-year-old City girl'. She works for the Depop vintage clothing app in London. 'My life was turned upside down three years ago when I started taking the pill again after a five-year break. After about three months back on Microgynon I started to notice a feeling of burning and really bad irritation. It felt like I had fibreglass in my pants.' Three years later, Suzie is still in pain, after being diagnosed with vulvodynia, which the NHS defines as 'persistent, unexplained pain in the vulva . . . Vulvodynia can become a long-term problem that's very distressing to live with,'[22] they add, helpfully.

The NHS solutions are 'lifestyle changes' like avoiding scented soaps and even putting Vaseline on your vulva if you go swimming in chlorinated water. There are also suggestions of anaesthetic gel, lube, antidepressants and cognitive behavioural therapy, which may help if there's been psychological or physical trauma. The prestigious Mayo clinic in America is equally vague: 'Vulvodynia (vul-voe-DIN-e-uh) is a type of long-term pain or discomfort around the outer part of the female genitals, called the vulva. It lasts at least three months and has no clear cause.' Wait a minute. Why is there no mention of low estrogen or hormonal contraception as a possible contribution to the problem on either advice site?

The first doctor Suzie went to did not even look at her painful vulva, and prescribed antibiotics for a urinary tract infection that she also had. Suzie spent a year and a half searching for answers on the NHS, and someone even suggested she should get her vagina Botoxed to avoid the pain, but it was only when she paid for a private consultant that she got an answer: she had 'hormonally mediated vulvodynia', and she should stop the progestin-only contraception pill. 'There was an immediate reduction in pain, and she also prescribed a topical combined estrogen and testosterone cream. Three years ago I was at 8 on the pain scale, and now I'm nearer to 4 or 5.' She thinks her pain receptors have been permanently damaged. Suzie's partner was 'very, very understanding' over the three years and they are still together. 'For a while having a sex life depended on whether I could handle the pain, but I potentially will have to live for ever with the side effects of the pill.'

Why are doctors so ill-informed about vulvodynia? There is plenty of information out there. In 2021, a round-up concluded that hormonal contraception caused a double-pronged attack on women sensitive to certain progestins, by lowering estrogen levels in the vulva causing pain, and lowering free testosterone in the brain.[23] The combination was 'a vicious circle', and there was no guessing which women on the pill would suffer from vulvodynia – it could be a genetic predisposition.

There is also a newer preparation, made with DHEA (dehydroepiandrosterone), which is the natural hormone precursor to estrogen and testosterone in your body. The vaginal pessary brand is IntraRosa in the US and UK, generically known as prasterone, and it had significant improvements of vaginal dryness and pain,[24] perhaps because it works with the many testosterone receptors as well as the estrogen receptors in the vulva. Yes, our ladyparts are full of supposedly male hormone receptors. I can vouch for DHEA too; I had a humdinger of a urinary tract infection when I dehydrated last summer. I had to take antibiotics, which killed the infection, but they knocked out my vaginal microbiome in the process. It was dry and painful, and I used IntraRosa for a week, and returned to normal – much better than the estrogen-only pessaries I'd previously been prescribed.

The new generation of contraceptive pills, which contain body-identical estrogen instead of the older synthetic ethinylestradiol, seem to perform better for mental health, and it turns out they have a more positive effect on sex lives too. One of these pills is called Drovelis in the UK and Nextstellis in the US, and it contains estetrol, a copy of one of the four natural estrogens we make. (This one is an estrogen produced by babies during pregnancy.) In a small 2023 trial of around a hundred women given three different combined contraceptive combinations – ethinylestradiol and levonorgestrel (Microgynon type), ethinylestradiol and drospirenone (Yasmin type) and estetrol and drospirenone (Drovelis) – those on the Drovelis pill had lower increases in sex hormone binding globulins (SHBG) compared to the Yasmin and Microgynon type pills. So, women's free testosterone stayed higher on Drovelis. That body-identical pill also had less impact on lowering DHEA levels (testosterone and estrogen precursors), so it was better for vaginal lubrication. (There's one caveat here – the trial was approved and published in the *Journal of Sexual Medicine*[25] but a grant for the work came from Mithra, the manufacturers of Drovelis.) But in general, we know from hormone-deprived women in menopause that both trans-dermal and vaginal body-identical estrogens help improve dry vulvas and lower UTIs.

Another pill, under the brands Lafamme, Natazia and Qlaira, contains the body-identical estrogen estra-diol valerate and the progestin dienogest and is different because its changing hormone levels mimic women's nat-ural cycles, with a 28-day packet containing four dummy pills for a short bleed and a reduced hormone-free inter-val. In a small trial of fifty-seven women,[26] most reported better scores on a quality-of-life questionnaire at three months and fewer problems with sex. By the sixth month, desire, arousal, orgasm, enjoyment and sexual activity improved. These body-identical pills are never a first offer-ing from doctors as they are more expensive, but they are worth asking for and trying out.

A third pill, Zoely, also contains body-identical estrogen and the progestin nomegestrol acetate (NOMAC), and again seems to show better performance. NOMAC does not bind to sex hormone binding globulin,[27] so it does not lower free testosterone. In a tiny but highly entertaining study, a bunch of Italian scientists measured the Clitoral Doppler Ultrasound of ten women on Zoely. (Who knew there even was a Clitoral Doppler Ultrasound?) They assessed the clitoris's 'pulsatility index', which reflects resistance to blood flow and found that women on Zoely were scoring better – or perhaps throbbing more? – than those on older oral contraceptives. Enjoy.

WHAT REALLY IS LIBIDO?

It is abundantly clear that hormonal contraception can cause a negative impact on female libido, but predicting precisely what will happen is almost anyone's guess, depending on each woman, and the composition of each pill. We know that most progestins can lower our testosterone levels, and that estrogen deprivation leaves vaginas high and dry. Healthcare professionals in contraception often make much of the complexity of libido, and how it is profoundly affected by other variables, like relationships and trauma. That's absolutely true, but if we can get the mechanics and hormonal chemistry right, better sex may follow. I'm thinking of all the women who have written to me, who lost years and even decades of pleasure to the pill and were gaslighted about their symptoms.

I want to conclude by thinking about the libido itself, and something I heard from Dr Dan Reisel of University College London, who is, unusually, trained in neuroscience and gynaecology. We were at a medical conference, and behind Dr Reisel was a screen showing a giant female brain lit up with testosterone and estrogen receptors. He was explaining that testosterone was neither a female nor a male hormone, but both, and how it can convert to estrogen too. He was discussing the proven effect of top-up testosterone gel in improving the sex lives of menopausal women with flatlining hormones,[28] and the fact that testosterone affects our energy, mental sharpness, mood, bones and muscles too.

At the moment, the NHS only prescribes testosterone to women for low libido, but Dr Reisel pointed out that the word libido, when it was coined by the early psychotherapist Sigmund Freud, meant far more than just sex. Freud wrote: 'Libido is an expression taken from the theory of the emotions. We call by that name the energy . . . of those instincts which have to do with all that may be comprised under the word "love".' For Freud, libido meant sexual love, family love, 'friendship and love for humanity in general, and also devotion to concrete objects and to abstract ideas.'[29] Libido is literally a life force. What else are we taking away from women when we suppress their libidos and their testosterone with the contraceptive pill?

CHAPTER FIVE

YOUR BRAIN ON THE PILL

At a laboratory in Newcastle, around a hundred young heterosexual female university students are sniffing sweaty T-shirts in the name of science. These T-shirts have been worn for two nights in a row by perspiring, smelly men — or 'odour donors' — who were paid a tenner for their efforts. Our female sniffers are either on the contraceptive pill, or not, and are being paid £25 for their three months of commitment. They will rate the shirts for 'pleasantness', inhaling the scent through a 'nose hole' in a large jar containing the T-shirt. The results were fascinating. It turned out that the pill-users were more likely to select the smells of men who have immune system genes closer to their own, while those cycling naturally were attracted by the pheromones of men with very different immunity — even when they were already in a steady relationship.[1] In essence, pill-users seemed to like a 'brother' type and non-users like the 'other', someone with very different genes from their own.

Professor Craig Roberts, instigator of this experiment, said he believed that: 'On the pill, your hormonal state mimics pregnancy, with high progesterone levels, so you tend to look for kin, someone who will help you with the baby.' Or perhaps it is just the steady levels of progestin that keep women calm. 'Off the pill women tend to choose someone very different from them, so their offspring will have a good mix of immune system genes,' he said. It's outbreeding rather than inbreeding. To make the preferences clearer, Professor Roberts and his team also tested the same group of women before they started taking the pill, and three months later, and their preferences changed when on hormonal contraception. 'The pill is having an effect. It's subtle but detectable. What are the consequences of that downstream?' he asked.

DOES THE PILL AFFECT SEXUAL ATTRACTION?

Is this a big deal or not? It certainly is on TikTok, where misreporting of the science has the anti-pill brigade suggesting that humankind is breeding with the wrong sort of person after hormonal contraception, and our mass immunity will be compromised for ever. Since only around 12 per cent of women are on the pill, we will probably survive as a species. But perhaps it's worth taking a break from the pill to test your real, unmedicated self out before committing to becoming a future parent? And let's be clear, people fancy people for all sorts of reasons other than their smell, like being a billionaire or having a highly developed sense of irony. Plus, there are all sorts of caveats here, not least from Professor Roberts, who is now in the Division of Psychology at the University of Stirling. He points out there have been some studies that conflict with his conclusions. But in general, the evidence points to the synthetic hormones in the pill changing our behaviour, in small but possibly significant ways.

The T-shirt sniffing went on way back in 2008, but in 2013 Professor Roberts was also involved in an experiment where they found pill use changed women's preferences for more masculine features in men.[2] It was a small but fascinating window into how women choose their partners, or indeed one-night stands. The researchers recruited fifty-five women and tested them to see which faces they preferred. The tests used opposite-sex and same-sex faces manipulated using computer graphics techniques to appear more or less masculine. Then eighteen of the women volunteered to go on the contraceptive pill for three months, while thirty-seven stayed on natural cycles. Three months in, the pill-users had a significantly decreased preference for male facial masculinity, but their preferences for same-sex faces remained the same.

The researchers also looked at 170 partners of another group of women who had started relationships while on the pill and discovered that the pill-users' partners tended to have less masculine faces than partners of women on natural cycles. Professor Roberts explained that many studies have shown that women prefer more masculine, symmetrical and genetically unrelated men during ovulation compared with the rest of their cycle. 'Those monthly changes in preferences might have had evolutionary benefits in terms of reproductive success,' he said. Do visual clues matter even more now that so many of us instinctively swipe on Tinder, Bumble, Hinge and other dating sites? Will our changing preferences for masculine facial architecture cause humanity to evolve differently?

CAN WOMEN BE ON HEAT?

There has been a surprising amount of international research into the effects of ovulation and hormonal contraception on sexual attraction, and some of the small studies are quite fascinating, in particular this one from the journal *Evolution and Human Behavior*, done by three male scholars in 2007: 'Ovulatory cycle effects on tip earnings by lap dancers: economic evidence for human estrus?'[3] Yes, the researchers asked professional lap dancers to keep a record of their nightly tip earnings for two months and tabulated that with their menstrual cycles and contraceptive pill use. The dancers received $67 per hour when they were near ovulation, 'on heat', so to speak, but only $52 at less fertile times, and a mere $37 when on their periods. Pill-users had no mid-cycle uplift in tip earnings, and they made only $193 per shift on average compared to normally cycling women making $276 – a loss of more than US $80 per shift to hormonal contraception.

'Because academics may be unfamiliar with the gentlemen's club subculture, some background may be helpful to understand why this is an ideal setting for investigating real-world attractiveness effects of human female estrus,' advised the researchers. They went on to explain that the women they were studying worked in the lap-dancing clubs of Albuquerque, New Mexico. The routines involved dancing topless and wearing bikini bottoms on stage, but the dancers' main earnings came from tips when sitting on men's knees in the audience, usually for the length of a three-minute song. The workers were paid $30 to log their cycles and tips, and a graph shows pill-users consistently lagging behind on earnings (they seemed to have chosen to have bleeds on the pill too). There were only eighteen dancers in the study, so looks and stage abilities may have influenced earnings too.

While the lap-dancing analysis may be of limited, if entertaining, use, it turns out that many studies show men's testosterone rising when the signals from women's ovulation set it off. Women's estrogen levels peak at ovulation, and their testosterone perks up a bit too, so everyone is on a hormonal high. It's time to get out the smelly T-shirts again, and this time it is ovulating women who are doing the overnight sweating and men who are doing the sniffing in this 'Scent of a Woman' study from Florida State University.[4] 'Men exposed to the scent of an ovulating woman subsequently displayed higher levels of testosterone than did men exposed to the scent of a non-ovulating woman or a control scent. Hence, olfactory cues signalling women's levels of reproductive fertility were associated with specific endocrinological responses in men; responses that have been linked to sexual behaviour and the initiation of romantic courtship.'

Basically, we are all on heat. Well, except perhaps in Scandinavian countries, where researchers looked at the hormone levels of Swedish couples[5] and did not see a general increase in male testosterone when that man's partner ovulated. But perhaps the hormonal leaps happen more when we are out on the hunt for strangers? The effect does seem to occur across nations. A study in Nagasaki, Japan,[6] this time using the separate backs and fronts of T-shirts worn by women, found that 'the odour emitted from the backs of women in the ovulatory phase was found to increase testosterone secretion in men, whereas the odour emitted from the chests of women in the ovulatory phase reduced cortisol secretion [an indicator of stress] in men.' Sexy — and relaxing.

And finally, in the hunter/huntress stakes, another burning scientific question: does hormonal contraception affect the amount of make-up you wear? Investigators recruited thirty-six students at the University of Grenoble in Spain and asked them how much time they spent putting on make-up. 'We found that women not using the contraceptive pill (i.e. naturally cycling women) reported spending more time applying cosmetics for an outing than did women who use the contraceptive pill.[7] We also found that the faces of these naturally cycling women were rated [by others] as wearing more cosmetics than the faces of the women using the contraceptive pill. Thus, we found clear associations between contraceptive pill use and make-up use.' This could be a load of codswallop since those on the pill were perhaps already having more regular sex, and those not on it were enthusiastically out on the pull slathered in lip gloss. But perhaps it's another little indication of the mysterious ways of hormonal contraception.

'COMING OFF CONTRACEPTION TURNED ME QUEER'

All these studies are set in the cis heterosexual world, and since the research is presently lacking, the effect of pill use on changing sexual attraction for lesbian, trans and non-binary people is anyone's guess. There was, however, a headline that caught my roving eye in PinkNews: 'Woman claims coming off contraception turned her queer — and now she could not be happier.'[8] The story was of thirty-year-old Tessa Bona from Melbourne, Australia, who went on the pill aged fifteen. She only ever dated men and came off the pill for the first time when she broke up with her long-term boyfriend. Within a few weeks she said: 'Everything changed . . . I felt like an entirely different person.' She started going out with women, and said she is now bisexual but more attracted to women. 'It's actually hilarious. The sexual attraction to guys is pretty much all gone.' At the time of the report, she had been with her new female partner Phoebe for six months and declared it was 'love at first sight', adding 'it breaks my heart to think this might never have happened if I was still on the pill.' I can only offer you details of romance, not science here, but I expect a young researcher somewhere will be lining up the T-shirts for LGBTQI+ sniffing soon.

DOES THE PILL AFFECT LONG-TERM MATE PREFERENCE?

Back in cavewoman times, we may have been in the habit of improving our gene pool by grabbing the tall, handsome hunter for a quick shag and procreation, but settling down with the shorter, sensible gatherer in the long term – and the gatherer would never know he wasn't the father. Have that in mind as we return to Professor Roberts' team in 2012,[9] which conducted a study of the long-term relationships of hundreds of Czech couples. Some couples got together on the pill, others while naturally cycling. The researchers discovered that 'women who used oral contraception when they met their partner scored lower on measures of sexual satisfaction and partner attraction, experienced increasing sexual dissatisfaction during the relationship, and were more likely to be the one to initiate an eventual separation if it occurred.'

Professor Roberts explained that use of hormonal contraception 'may contribute to relationship outcome, with implications for human family cohesion and quality of life later on'. On the other hand, women who met their partner while on the pill 'were more satisfied with their partner's paternal provision, and thus had longer relationships and were less likely to separate'. Perhaps we make more sensible and practical long-term choices of partner on the pill, but there are also stories of women falling in love while on the pill, coming off it to start trying for a baby and finding their sexual attraction to their partner is waning.

The cavewoman-wants-hunter 'ovulatory shift hypothe-sis' is backed up by some experiments looking at women's attraction to men with more conventionally masculine and symmetrical features. This is the last time I'll men-tion smelly T-shirts, but at the peak of ovulation, women preferred the scent of shirts worn by symmetrical-featured men. At other times in their cycle, normally ovulating women and women on the pill showed no significant preference for either symmetrical or asymmetrical men's scent.[10] I also suspect that hormones and pheromones are minor factors in the big relationship picture, but I am feeling secretly relieved that I met my partner a couple of years before he lost much of his sense of smell after Covid. What effect is that loss having on pair bonding for so many people? Another study that looked at the amount of time ovulating and non-ovulating women spent looking at male faces showed that they spent no longer looking at either masculinised or feminised faces.[11] When asked to pick a potential long-term partner, they stared at the men for longer.

YOUR BRAIN CONTROLLED BY BIRTH CONTROL

The popular doyenne of the brain-on-birth-control move-ment is Dr Sarah E. Hill, a social psychologist at Texas Christian University, who has written a book, *How the Pill Changes Everything: Your Brain on Birth Control*. She discusses the effect of hormonal contraception in detail, and makes this suggestion: 'There's no need for alarm, but . . . if you meet your partner when you are on the pill, it probably can't hurt to see how you feel about your partner when you are off the pill before making anything permanent.'[12] She points out that 'the brain and the rest of the body are too flush with hormone receptors for the pill *not* to change women.' There are changes in areas of the brain responsible for 'emotional processing, social interactions, attention, learning, memory, facial recognition, self-control, eating behaviour and language processing. And we're also talking about non-brain body parts like the immune system, the stress response and your gut hormones.'[13]

I talked to Dr Hill about her upcoming research into alcohol consumption and pill use, and she explained that pill use lowers levels of a neurosteroid called allopregnanolone, which stimulates GABA [gamma-aminobutyric acid] pleasure receptors in our brains.'[14] Stimulating these receptors slows our brains down, making us less anxious and more relaxed. 'When GABA is low, women tend to take matters into their own hands and have a drink,' she said. Her laboratory has also been looking into the degree to which people enjoy music on the pill, after Dr Hill found her own enthusiasm for music returned when she went natural after years on the pill. In tests, oral contraception users rated a variety of musical clips with lower scores compared to non-users. Alert Spotify.

In the last decade, a vast new academic field has opened up in the neuroscience of hormonal contraceptives, and it's fascinating. Neuroscientists want to empower women with information about the biopsychological effects of the pill, with more rigorous randomized controlled trials, because existing research is limited. 'Studies nonetheless highlight that the effects of hormonal contraceptives on the nervous system are complex and can vary because of individual differences, contraceptive type and formulation, and timing of use, among other factors."[15]

One of the leading researchers in the field is Professor Belinda Pletzer, a neuroscientist at the University of Salzburg in Austria. She discovered that women on hormonal contraception had a smaller amount of grey matter in the hippocampus area of the brain, which has a role in learning and memory.[16] Unlike previous research, Professor Pletzer decided not just to look at how the pill affected the brain, but how different progestins specifically changed matters, masculinising and feminising the brain just as they do the body in terms of hairiness or breast size. Her team found that anti-androgenic progestins promoted larger grey matter volumes in areas connected to facial recognition, and androgenic progestins made it smaller.[17] In general, women are better at facial recognition than men, but increasing androgenic progestins means we lessen that feminine skill. (I have terrible facial recognition skills, and in one of my past lives I was a film critic. Disaster. I am also hopeless at introducing people at parties.) But in an upside for androgenic pill-users, the neuroscientists also found those women had a slight increase in grey matter involved with memory retrieval, motor skills and balance, compared to women not on contraception. There are also studies showing pill-users have reduced accuracy in recognising emotions compared to naturally cycling women.[18] But maybe that more masculine attitude works for some women, particularly those doing tough jobs.

These brain changes are tiny in the big scheme of things, but perhaps a change in pill might bring an edge in chess or maths or architecture for someone. Some studies have shown that more androgenic progestins seemed to slightly increase spatial ability, but the synthetic estrogen ethinylestradiol diminished spatial performance. Rats who were given the anti-androgenic progestin drospirenone had good spatial working memory in a maze, but when they added ethinylestradiol, those benefits were reversed.[19] Worth thinking about around exam time if you're on Yasmin, which contains these ingredients. That's probably a bonkers idea, but these minor changes are clear signs that every pill is very different and complex, and there may be very good reasons to swap brand.

THE PILL BLUNTS NATURAL RESPONSE TO STRESS

Pill-taking women have a blunted free-cortisol response to stress compared to naturally cycling women or men, as though they have experienced chronic stress over a long time. Being with other people is one of the most effective ways of reducing stress, but a recent study found that social activities like playing board games or singing songs reduced stress hormone levels in naturally cycling women, but had no effect on women on the pill.[20] Natural progesterone is broken down into the hormone allopregnanolone, which is involved in a wide range of calming effects and can influence the stress response — but synthetic progestin does not. That said, one synthetic progestin, Nestorone,[21] has been shown to have all sorts of positive neuroprotective and anti-inflammatory effects, including increasing calming neurons, and was able to decrease the neurological disability and increase the motor behaviour in animals, which might even help patients with multiple sclerosis. Nestorone needs to be taken transdermally and is available in a vaginal ring – and it's been selected as the progestin element in the new trials of a male contraceptive gel. Gentlemen first.

Dr Caitlin Taylor studies the effects of oral contraception using MRI brain imaging at the Jacobs Lab at the University of California in Santa Barbara, and she gave me an overview of the field. 'I am still filled with total indignation, wondering how has this pill been around for sixty years, and we've only just started asking these questions? We have ignored this for too long, we have not seen this as a worthy question, but it is a messy area to grapple with. And I do understand why we're not finding all the answers right away.'

Part of the problem is the inconsistency of study findings, using dozens of different hormonal contraceptives and not necessarily differentiating them. Dr Taylor is working with other scientists to establish and grow a huge neuroimaging database – part of the Ann S. Bowers Women's Brain Health Initiative – that is designed with women's health in mind. 'It's not going to be only women. Once that database is available to a larger global scientific audience, we are hoping that they will be able to mine the data to ask the questions that we were not able to ask because this dataset didn't exist.' The scientists will look at brains when women have PMS or postnatal depression or are menopausal or pregnant or post-pregnant. 'We will be capturing as many people as we can to cover the lifespan.' This is a wealth of data which may make a huge difference to women's contraceptive and hormonal choices in the future.

Dr Taylor has done some research scanning a woman's brain every day across a menstrual cycle, and then scanning her again for a month after she had been on the pill for a year. 'I found that across the menstrual cycle, there were certain parts of the hippocampus that changed in volume as her progesterone levels changed. And then I found that when she was on the pill, I no longer saw those volume changes across the same time period. And what was interesting is that in her case, she was taking a formulation of the pill that was low dose enough that it actually didn't suppress her estrogen, but it only suppressed progesterone. So when progesterone was replaced by a progestin, we no longer saw these volume effects.'

'WE ARE WORTHY OF STUDY'

There is so much to discover. We know these synthetic hormones suppress our own production of those hormones – to some extent – but does the brain sometimes see synthetic hormones as an extra supply, something steadying, or just treat them completely differently? And how does that change the structure of the brain over ten or even twenty years? 'We also don't know what happens in a developing brain across puberty when adolescents are being prescribed the pill. Girls are starting at fairly young ages while the brain is still developing, which is a huge hormonal transition period.' Dr Taylor notes that research has mostly just focused on the reproductive success of the pill, and not considered the systemic effect. 'It's often used as a BandAid for adolescents' problems, when we should be investigating the underlying condition, like PCOS.'

Dr Taylor also understands that women are stopping the pill because they are concerned about these effects, but we still can't provide them with full information. 'There was the assumption for ever that because women have these cycling hormones, we would add too much noise to the scientific data. So they just studied men and male animals and extrapolated from that. Our hormones do not make us messier or noisier than males, and this is finally being addressed. I don't think male scientists were interested, so it just went under the radar until we had women who were able to enter the scientific field and ask questions that were relevant to their previous experiences,' said Dr Taylor. 'We are worthy of study.'

I feel like we are just scratching the surface here in terms of the myriad effects hormonal contraception may have on the brain, particularly when you think that female brains are packed with estrogen, progesterone and testosterone receptors. How crazy was it to assume for decades that the pill just switched our ovaries off, or plumped up our cervical mucus, when it was running wild in our heads? The longer we use the pill, the more profound the changes seem to be, and maybe some of us want those steadier, more masculine mindsets. We also see through the latest studies of cross-sex hormones in trans people that the brain can change profoundly. While the tech bros are playing with 'nootropics' – supposed neurological enhancers – women may also one day play with their brain hormones. But first, we need solid, long-term evidence of the effect of hormonal contraception on the brain, and not just the tiny studies above.

CHAPTER SIX

THE COIL

At Port Askaig on the Scottish island of Islay in January, it was pishing with rain, cold and dark. Dr Sally Darnborough was in her car in the queue for the evening ferry back to the mainland in Argyll. She had about an hour to wait, and at last she had time to talk to me about what she'd been doing – fitting contraceptive coils for the islanders. The ferry crossing is two hours, so she wouldn't get back home until almost midnight. But Dr Darnborough is dedicated to her work as an NHS GP and goes over every six weeks on the ferry to Islay (population 3,000) to fit intrauterine contraceptive devices as part of a one-stop contraception and women's health clinic.

Women want coils – and other contraceptive advice – and it's hard to find a trained coil fitter in rural areas. Dr Darnborough fits the two types of coils. The copper IUD or intrauterine device is hormone-free and alters the cervical mucus and also stops the egg implanting. The hormonal IUS intrauterine system (brands like Mirena) releases the progestin levonorgestrel, which thickens cervical mucus and inhibits implantation. In 2023, the waiting times for hormonal and copper coil fittings were as much as a year in parts of Devon and Northern Ireland, and from a week to six months across the rest of the country. Women are desperate, and sometimes the long wait for a coil ends in unintended pregnancy and abortion, according to MSI Reproductive Choices. In the US, Planned Parenthood said they had a 41 per cent increase in coil appointments since the abortion laws changed.[1] For pregnancy prevention, it's one of the safest bets, being 99 per cent effective.

Despite the internet algorithm, which emphasises the horror stories around the discomfort of coil fittings, the fact is that once they're in and settled – which can take months rather than the weeks mentioned in medical literature – the majority of women are very happy with the fit-and-forget convenience of coils. 'More and more women want coils, even the younger ones are hearing about it from their friends. We are prescribing the pill less, and more coils, but we can't get enough trained fitters,' said Dr Darnborough, as she moved up the ferry queue. 'You've got to pay for a course with the Faculty of Sexual and Reproductive Healthcare, and then fit at least seven under supervision. And keep up your qualification. Rural doctors do lots of other procedures all the time without so much bureaucracy. There aren't enough trainers and there's a bottleneck for people who want to get trained in coil fitting.' But she rolls up her sleeves and gets on with it. Who knew that people were sailing across lochs for coil fittings?

But women also come miles to Dr Darnborough on the Portavadie ferry from Cowal to her clinic in Tarbert for fittings, and she believes that local GPs and nurses would be keen to be trained in this so that women don't need to spend a day travelling. 'Most doctors can deal with smears, speculums, cervixes, so why not the coil?' she said. 'But what they need to learn is how to counsel someone and explain what happens so they are relaxed beforehand. I always have a nurse at the top end.' Dr Darnborough says it's important to manage women's expectations of what will happen post-insertion – so they feel confident. 'They need to understand the side effects, to expect cramps afterwards, and doctors need to know what to do for the few women who feel faint – it usually passes. It's so important women's fears about what happens are allayed – a verbal analgesic – since one woman who's had a bad experience will put dozens of people off, and most women have good experiences.' She also always uses a local anaesthetic beforehand – 'four squirts of Xylocaine does it'.

WHY DO WE HAVE A LOVE–HATE RELATIONSHIP WITH THE COIL?

For some older women, the dark shadow of the Dalkon Shield debacle hangs over considering the coil. The Dalkon Shield was a strange, crab-shaped coil used by over two million women in the UK and US in the early 1970s, and it was banned after it caused serious pelvic infections leading to infertility or even death. Unlike safer modern coils, the thread for pulling out the Dalkon was made of permeable material that harboured bacteria, and encouraged infection. The American Centers for Disease Control and Prevention put out research in 1973 on the risks of the Dalkon Shield, but it took until 1974 for the coil to be taken off the market by the A.H. Robins pharmaceutical company, and there was no product recall. So thousands of women were left at risk for years. Only in 1985, after 9,500 women's claims had been litigated or settled, did the company file for bankruptcy and set up a $2.3 billion trust fund to deal with the thousands of pending cases.[2] The neglect and dismissal of women's suffering is at the heart of this deeply shameful piece of contraceptive history, and I will explore that in depth in Chapter 12.

Present-day coils are made from different materials from the Dalkon, and have a good safety record. Dr Darnborough is very positive, but for many women, the coil is contraceptive Marmite. For every period-free, problem-free success story, there is also a tale of an agonising insertion, weird mood changes, or months of unresolved bleeding and cramps. But in the wider picture, seen in reviews of contraceptive methods by 5,000 users on The Lowdown,[3] the Mirena hormonal coil gets some of the highest ratings, at 3.6 out of 5, and women love the fact they can put it in for over five or more years and get on with their lives. The coil also lessens or stops periods for most women, and some non-binary people and trans men like it for the diminution of bleeding and because it's more discreet than a daily pill. All women still ovulate on the copper coil. Most women still ovulate on the hormonal coil, which can be good for mood and sex drive – in the first year, about 45 per cent ovulate and by four years in, it is 75 per cent.[4] Compared to a progestin-only pill, the hormonal coil releases around a tenth of the level of hormones daily, which can often be better tolerated. Only the fertility awareness method is rated higher than the coil at The Lowdown, but we know the pregnancy risks and daily hassle of that.

I've had three hormonal coils, and I wouldn't be where I am today without them. I've got one in now as I write. If you're thinking, by the way, that a coil actually looks like a coil or a Slinky, you'd be wrong. It's actually a three-centimetre-long T-shaped device that unfurls like a Lilliputian umbrella in your womb and exerts extraordinary change. Let's take an unbiased tour of the copper and hormonal coils, and hear about the good, the bad and the ugly experiences.

HOW THE DIFFERENT COILS WORK

The copper coil

The copper coil or intrauterine device (IUD) is hormone-free and made of plastic and copper, a metal which makes the womb and fallopian tubes toxic to sperm by causing an inflammatory reaction. In these unpleasant conditions, the sperm are no longer viable and can't fertilise an egg. This coil lasts for up to ten years and is also one of the most reliable forms of morning-after contraception, since it stops an egg from implanting. If you think you have slipped up the night before, you can make an emergency appointment at a sexual health clinic for a copper coil fitting (if you are lucky enough to live in a city that has that service).

The copper coil makes bleeding heavier for an estimated 40 per cent of women at the start usually in the first three to six months,[5] but this does get better over time, and women love being free of synthetic hormones. Useful tip: you can ask for one of the mini-coils (like the TT380 Slimline Mini), which are 23.2mm wide rather than 31.8mm, and shorter in length too – more comfortable for women with a smaller uterus or those who have not had children. The mini copper coils only last five years, but they are much better tolerated. In one small study of women, mostly in their twenties, only 15 per cent of those with the mini-coil asked for removal in the year following due to pain and bleeding, compared to 32 per cent of those with the larger coil.[6] Other studies have shown a discontinuation rate of between 15 to 20 per cent for the copper coil. If you're already a flooder, like me and so many of us, the copper coil is worth avoiding and the hormonal coil may work better.

The hormonal coil

The hormonal coil tends to lighten periods over time, and almost half of women have no periods, or small irregular ones, within two years.[7] That's why hormonal coils are often prescribed for women struggling with heavy bleeding. This contraception is known as the intrauterine system (IUS), and the hormonal coils include the Mirena, Levosert and Benilexa at 32mm width, and the slightly smaller, lower-dose Kyleena and Jaydess at 28mm, which are often easier to fit in smaller wombs. It is worth asking specially for a smaller version if you have not had children. They all contain the same synthetic progestin hormone, levonorgestrel, which is released in tiny amounts every day.

There is no or little risk of blood clots with the hormonal coil, unlike the pill, but the small breast cancer risk seems to be much the same as the pill[8] and increases with longer use and age. Hormonal coils last for over five years, apart from the Jaydess, which works for three. There's a slightly increased risk of ectopic (tubal) pregnancies with the lower-dose coils. Because the coil is in the womb where the action is, a lower dose of hormones is enough to prevent pregnancy, and the Mirena starts by delivering 20mcg per day of levonorgestrel, decreasing to about 10mcg by five years. This is much lower than the 'low-dose' contraceptive pill. For both types of coil, there is also a back-up 'foreign body reaction', which increases inflammation and makes it difficult for the embryo to implant in the womb.

ME AND MY MIRENA

As a card-carrying coil user, I'm on my third Mirena and very happy with it. (They really do give you a card to keep at the doctors', which notes the serial number and the date of insertion.) I got my coils put in by great health care professionals without any numbing gel or anaesthetic. On each occasion, it was painful for a minute or two, and I had cramps on the day and for a few weeks afterwards, but that was it. (I now realise, after dozens of women sent their painful coil-fitting stories in to me on my @pillscandal Instagram, that I was lucky; more about the trials of insertion later.) I've had a couple of coils for contraception when I was fertile, and now I use one as the progestin element of my hormone replacement therapy. The coil has no negative effect on my mood or libido; it just sits there quietly getting on with the job.

When you top up your depleted estrogen after menopause, you need to balance it with a synthetic progestin or body-identical progesterone, so your womb lining doesn't get too thick and put you at risk of serious bleeding or uterine cancer. The coil also helps to reduce bleeding from fibroids, which is great if, like me and the majority of menopausal and many other women, you have a few.[9] When I was still having periods, the Mirena didn't stop the flow at all. I still needed super-plus tampons, but I suppose it might have prevented absolutely gargantuan bleeds, which 44 per cent of women experience in their forties due to hormone fluctuations in the perimenopause.[10] I've had my Mirenas replaced after every five years on NHS advice, but now I've researched this book I've discovered they last *up to eight years* for contraception, according to the latest guidance.[11] Why weren't we told that? And how much money has the manufacturer made by everyone underestimating the use-by date for years?

WHY DO WE REACT DIFFERENTLY TO THE SAME HORMONES IN THE COIL AND THE PILL?

What interests me here is how differently we react to the same progestin in different parts of our bodies. As I mentioned earlier, I felt flat and had low libido on Microgynon, the pill containing 150mcg of levonorgestrel, but I feel absolutely fine with the 10-20mcg being delivered locally to my womb by my Mirena coil. That's probably because, unlike the oral progestin in the pill, the progestin in the coil is not being processed in my stomach and my liver first, before it reaches my cervix and womb. The correlation between a lower dose and lesser side effects has been seen in research on the pill too,[12] although a minority of women sensitive to progestins can still get a bad reaction.

The different method of delivery – but the same progestin, levonorgestrel – also worked for my daughter, Molly, who felt depressed on Rigevidon but did much better mentally on the low-dose Kyleena coil, apart from months of painful cramping. When I went with Molly for an ultrasound scan to check her coil was in the right place (it was), I saw for the first time how tiny a non-pregnant womb is: about four or five centimetres wide and seven centimetres long, like a smallish pear. I expressed my doubts that this pear-thing could ever expand to hold a seven-pound baby, which I had seen on my own pregnancy ultrasounds. 'Think of it like a deflated football,' said the gynaecologist helpfully, scanning away. I still find it strange that we are so ignorant about this womb, this organ of creation and destruction, unseen and all powerful. It helps to be able to imagine your coil in place.

SIDE EFFECTS OF THE COIL

Unsurprisingly, the side effects reported by women using the copper coil on sites like The Lowdown and social media are more problematic than those studied in scientific research papers, and obviously if you've had a bad experience, there is an incentive to go online to report it and warn others. TikTok is a junkyard of coil horror stories, with very few good experiences to balance it up. In one large-scale scientific study, 67 per cent said they had menstrual side effects,[13] but Lowdowners reported that 78 per cent had period-like cramps (normal for a few months) and 46 per cent had vaginal discharge, and they also had problems with lower back pain, breast tenderness and thrush. Dr Darnborough said it was worth warning that for some women after any kind of coil fitting, cramps could last on and off for six weeks, so they knew what to expect.

For both kinds of coils, there is a divide here between short term, settling-in side effects, and longer-term problems. Women should be better informed about both. Katharine Gale, an independent nurse consultant living in Wales who has fitted thousands of coils, said, 'We can't just say "take a paracetamol", we need to talk about the range of aftermath experiences: cramping can be for days, but also for weeks. Sometimes the uterus cramps to enable the coil to settle down and find a natural position.' On

The Lowdown, 61 per cent reported period-like cramps, 44 per cent tender breasts, 43 per cent vaginal discharge, 29 per cent lower back pain and 26 per cent breast enlargement. Lots of these diminish with time for most women. Of course, there are good side effects too: the hormonal coil can ease the symptoms of adenomyosis, endometriosis, fibroids and heavy painful periods. The US Food and Drug Administration coil summary[14] says that 23 per cent get decreased uterine bleeding, and 18 per cent no bleeding at all (amenhorrea). On the negative side, 16 per cent get headaches or migraines, 10 per cent get vulvovaginitis (inflammation of the vulva), 8 per cent breast pain, 6 per cent acne (levonorgestrel is an androgenic hormone) and 6 per cent get depressive mood. So, after the initial cramp-fest, most women find the coil comfortable, but you can see from the widely varying statistics and reports that there are all sorts of ways it can go wrong for the minority. Let's listen to those women.

When the hormonal coil plays havoc with your mental health

Anna Robertson is forty-one and now works as a midwife in south-west Scotland. When we talked, she was the picture of confidence and mental health, with her pink T-shirt, bouncing ponytail, and summer garden behind her – but the coil was her undoing. Anna had tried the pill and the contraceptive injection over the years, and was not happy with either. After she'd given birth to her second son a few years ago, she had a Mirena coil put in. 'That was awful, horrendous. I felt like I'd lost my mind.

It changed my behaviour, it made me reckless and me and my husband almost ended up splitting up. I felt like I'd had a personality transplant.'

As so often happens, women blame themselves and their circumstances and not their hormones. Anna must have been exceptionally sensitive to the levonorgestrel progestin in the coil; studies show progestin-only contraception seems to create a greater propensity for depressive disorders in vulnerable women.[15] Also, her middle son was diagnosed with cystic fibrosis, so she was dealing with a child with chronic illness as well as a new baby. The coil was in for five months and she was still bleeding erratically. 'This was driving me mental. I find it really hard to tolerate bleeding, but the doctor told me to give it six months. I just didn't feel right.' Her skin was bad, too, thanks to the progestin, and she went back on the drug Roaccutane for acne, which can also lower mood.

'I just didn't feel listened to, but I kept the contraception in, as I didn't want to have another baby. I see that all the time in my job.' From Anna's own experience, she knows how rarely even professionals connect contraceptive use with mental health. 'I was eighteen months with the coil. I was like a bear with a sore paw, and ready to leave my husband.' She was getting ready to move out with her sons when she got the coil taken out and she felt normal again within weeks. Anna and her husband are still together. 'Getting rid of it saved my marriage.'

Anna is now on Eloine, a low-dose pill similar to Yasmin with synthetic estrogen and drospirenone progestin, which is not androgenic and keeps acne at bay. She's happy with her contraception and not having any periods. (She is very annoyed that no one told her when she was younger that there was no need to bleed on the pill and that she could have taken it back-to-back without a monthly hormonal dip.) Her struggle with the coil has had one positive aspect: she started midwifery training in 2017 and loves it. 'It's fabulous to empower women with information and listen to them so they can find their own way. Women are so disempowered about knowing about their own bodies.'

Ironically, one of her jobs as a midwife is to discuss post-natal contraception with her pregnant patients and at the six-week check after birth. 'We're told to push them to get an implant or coil in.' But now Anna is more aware of shared decision-making with the patient. 'If someone makes a choice we don't agree with as professionals – we might think it's reckless, irresponsible, who does she think she is? But we always need to remember that sometimes women know what suits them. Health literacy is so important. Women need the language and tools to engage with the health system and ask for what they want.'

Can the coil sometimes cause anxiety and even panic attacks?

Here's another rare side effect you don't hear much about: panic attacks. Although there is now some medical literature on adverse progestin drug reactions causing panic attacks and anxiety,[16] there are only women self-reporting around the non-hormonal copper coil. But if you have high levels of copper in your body already, which has been linked to anxiety,[17] perhaps the addition of more is a risk?

I was talking to Charlotte Highmore, an account director in healthcare change, and she happened to mention she had decided to get the copper coil to avoid putting hormones into her body, but found there were other consequences: 'At first I bled for about sixteen weeks. I just thought that was what happened, and I got terrible cramps. But when I'd get a cramp, it would kick off a panic attack, so I got the copper coil out. I changed over to the Mirena Coil, the panic attacks disappeared, and I was absolutely fine.'

In one analysis of the GPs' database, 18 per cent reported an increased risk of anxiety on the coil and 22 per cent increased sleep problems.[18] On The Lowdown, 31 per cent said the hormonal coil had affected their mood, but that compared to 62 per cent on the combined pill. So that result is *not too bad* in the compromised world of contraception. So many struggle on, when perhaps they should track or journal their symptoms over weeks, and work out whether there are significant changes in mood.

After getting a low-dose Jaydess coil, journalist Olivia Petter, aged twenty-nine, knew something was wrong when she burst into tears seeing the word 'Walthamstow' lit up on the tube destination board – just because she had previously lived there. 'This was the latest in a series of strange emotional outbursts . . . Panic attacks had become a daily occurrence, as had four-hour binges of reality TV, and by December I couldn't remember the last day I hadn't cried. Then came thoughts I won't repeat,' she wrote in the *Sunday Times*.[19] 'Eventually my brain became completely consumed by darkness and on Christmas Eve I rang the Samaritans.'

Olivia had never experienced depression or anxiety before, and she began to suspect the synthetic hormones were the culprit. She went to her GP and said, 'I think my coil is making me mad.' He suggested it was just because she had moved house after a break-up. But Olivia insisted he take it out. 'My mood improved almost instantly – and I haven't had any mental health scares since.'

With equal unpredictability, some people have reported a phenomenon called a 'Mirena Crash', when women who are happily on the coil have psychological issues after the removal of the device and the loss of a steady stream of progestin. But the stories are anecdotal. Like so much in the contraceptive arena, no research into this currently exists.

FEARS AROUND COIL FITTING . . . AND REMOVAL

If you are going to have a coil fitted, it's best to know in detail exactly what happens and exactly what to ask for, so that there are no unpleasant surprises. Three-quarters of women in one study said the insertion procedure went 'very well' even though they coped with 'moderate to severe pain'.[20]

Fear and tension make pain worse; knowledge reduces it. Like many aspects of women's health, we all kept calm and carried on for years, not complaining about the pain of coil insertion or the aftermath, but in the UK in 2021, there was an eruption of stories from angry women who had been refused any anaesthetic during fitting or treated carelessly by medical staff. A conversation started on social media and went viral — as did one American woman's video later on TikTok, where she removed the coil herself because she could not get an appointment.[21] (Self-removal is an incredibly bad idea, as there's a risk of tearing or sepsis.) On my Instagram, one woman in York said she had waited a year for coil removal. Another said: 'I waited over two years to have my Mirena coil removed. No one would remove it!'[22] One doctor wrote of her own coil fitting: 'I paid so I could have anaesthetic. The one I had in a sexual health clinic was so painful I couldn't go through with it again.'[23] Stories also poured into me from women who had experienced extreme pain, or of fainting and panicking.

A typical message was this: 'I'm on my second coil, it was one of the last options for dealing with endometriosis, but it's really worked for me. However, my replacement Mirena inserted a few years ago (mid Covid) was one of the most painful experiences of my life, despite an experienced and wonderful gynae. My first coil wasn't great, but they offered me gas and air, but during Covid there was nothing, not even a nurse to hold my hand and reassure me . . . you bet on my third Mirena coil I will not go through that experience again. I feel there are constant lies told to women about painful gynae procedures. The "just take a paracetamol and you'll be fine" narrative has to change.'[24]

Dr Darnborough said women occasionally faint or feel lightheaded during the insertion, a 'vasovagal episode' that is usually harmless. Recovery requires additional time with the patient lying down, and then progressing slowly to sitting. Let's just look into that. Vasovagal syncope can happen due to stress during an injection, but in some coil fittings it's a sort of cervical shock, which results in a slow pulse rate, low blood pressure, and feeling sweaty or nauseated.[25] Wriggling your fingers and toes can help get the circulation moving again. Serious vasovagal episodes only happen to a few women, but it's worth hearing about beforehand, so you know it will pass. Most women have no idea about this, and it is absolutely clear that having teams of trained coil-fitters, with plenty of experience and a terrific bedside manner, could really help women feel more confident about asking for this very practical form of contraception. The NHS website, hoping not to put women off, plays down the difficulties: 'Let the person fitting your IUD know if you feel any pain or discomfort while you are having it fitted. You can ask to stop at any time. You can also take painkillers after having an IUD fitted if you need to. You may get period-type cramps afterwards, but painkillers can ease the cramps.'[26] You also need honest, more detailed advice from a health professional you trust who is, after all, about to put a foreign body into your body.

Partly because there was so much fear and loathing around the coil, despite its utility, we decided to try to diminish that fear when we made *Davina McCall's Pill Revolution* documentary for Channel 4 in 2023. Davina is a big proponent of the coil, having had them for years for contraception, and now for HRT, and in one of our early meetings she said: 'Why don't I get my next coil fitted on camera?' She checked with her teenage and twentysomething kids how they felt about that; go for it, they said. I was the producer of the film, and while we were interviewing the UK Women's Health Ambassador, Professor Dame Lesley Regan, we discovered not only was she fighting to have one-stop-shop women's health hubs set up round the country, but that she was also nicknamed 'Fairy Fingers' thanks to her coil-fitting abilities. Professor Regan agreed to fit the coil live on telly and talk us through it.

Davina lay down in the private One Welbeck Clinic with cameras focused on her face for reactions, and Professor Regan bustled in. (Let's be clear: you often get a far better patient experience, and guaranteed anaesthetic, in the private sector, as well as the luxury of time.) Professor Regan's bedside manner was simultaneously brisk and gentle, and she gave a step-by-step description of everything she did. First, she 'popped' some numbing anaesthetic gel, Instillagel, into the vagina. 'That'll feel a little bit cold, a little bit wet,' she advised. 'And where are you going on holiday this year?' Davina snorted with laughter. Professor Regan advised that the gel 'will help the speculum go in easily and it will also make the neck of the womb a little numb'. After insertion, Davina announced the speculum (which holds the vagina open) was 'not too bad. With this gel I barely feel a thing.' Then Professor Regan told Davina to take a deep breath and blow out sharply, and whipped the old coil out in a second, brandishing it in the air like a magician. 'That was a bit uncomfortable,' said Davina. 'I've got cramping like a period pain, but it's all quite handleable.'

Davina then got a numbing injection at either side of her cervix but didn't feel it due to the gel. The only really painful moment came when Professor Regan inserted a 'sound'— basically a thin measuring stick — up the cervix and into the womb to check the length, so the coil could be placed correctly. 'That felt like a scrape, like sharp period pains,' said Davina. But one deep breath later, the thin tube containing the furled coil went in, the T-shaped arms were released, and the coil was in the womb and the threads hanging down into the cervix (to check it is in place) were trimmed. Afterwards, there was just a little bit of pain in her lower abdomen. 'Ten minutes of discomfort is a small price to pay for five years of convenience,' said Davina. Then she took the tube home.

Davina's coil fitting was more like a cervical ballet, with numbing gel and an anaesthetic injection, as well as four decades of expertise from 'Fairy Fingers'. Most women do not get offered injections in the UK as they are usually only offered at sexual health clinics, but the NHS says women should be allowed to insist on a numbing gel; just make sure you ask or call beforehand. 'There are lots of measures we can take to minimise discomfort,' said Professor Regan. 'Take painkillers beforehand, and tell women exactly what's happening.'

She also spoke about the how the barriers to coil fitting training and waiting lists must change. The Faculty of Sexual Health and Reproductive Healthcare certifies coil fitters, and they have to be overseen by a registered trainer, who may not be available in areas, and the cost can be around £400 for doctors or nurses, as well as a time commitment on top of their day jobs. 'We need to improve access to training. It's not rocket science. This is basic maintenance, allowing you to get on with your life in a trouble-free way.'

Writing this chapter, I'm thinking what we need is the human equivalent of Kwik Fit tyre changes in the UK, or Jiffy Lube in America – experts who do one thing over and over, really well. You want someone like Professor Regan or Dr Darnborough who really knows their way round a womb and a cervix and the whole NHS health system. There was a time when it was much easier to get coils fitted in the UK, when GPs were paid extra by the government so long as they just *mentioned* LARCs – long-acting reversible contraceptives like the coil, injection or implant – during the consultation. Now that that payment has ended, so has many GPs' interest in keeping their coil training and expertise up to date, and a coil appointment takes longer, so is less profitable for the doctors' surgery group.

Practice makes perfect. Katharine Gale has fitted coils for years as a nurse and could probably do it in her sleep. Like many of us, she is both a patient and an activist, and sees the system from both sides. 'I feel like I've gone through the whole gynaecological textbook: I have endometriosis, I had a fibroid removed, I've had fertility treatment, I've had a son, and I walked out of my job as a matron at forty, with anxiety, depression and mental health symptoms – which turned out to be perimenopause, but it took me eighteen months to join up the dots.' She has a Mirena herself, aged forty-nine, to help manage her endometriosis pain and to hold the disease back from progressing. (The Endometriosis Society says coils have been shown to help with period pain, particularly for the first twelve to eighteen months.[27]) 'There is no real cure,' said Katharine. The coil also provides a two-for-one service, protecting her womb lining as she now takes Hormone Replacement Therapy. Even Katharine was on a two-month coil waiting list, where she lives in Lampeter; she had to travel to Aberystwyth to get it fitted. 'Couldn't you have fitted it yourself?' I asked with interest. She said it was probably better to get someone else.

Katharine also made a good point that coil fitting is shared decision making: 'If patients have had a painful experience before, I explain we'll try, but we can stop any time you want.' Women also fear perforation of the womb by the coil, a rare one in a thousand risk.[28] In all her years on fitting coils, Katharine has only had two incidences of perforations or tears (which often heal by themselves). 'One was due to a tiny uterus, another because the uterus had tissue separating it in the middle.' In most cases, what she can bring to the job is a detective's skill, an ability to feel what's going on in the vagina and womb, a bimanual vaginal examination. 'When you feel nothing, that's good; the womb is nice and small and normal. But if the womb feels really bulky and tender, that might be adenomyosis [tissue growing into the wall of the womb]. If someone's got endometriosis it will often feel fixed and stiff, and fibroids might make it feel bulky.'

What if we had nurses like Katharine everywhere, who are coil fitters, but can also tell you so much more about your womb? She was working fitting coils at a pilot community gynaecology service in North Bristol, but the funding to continue was cut. So, Katharine is now work-ing as a coach and runs a virtual menopause clinic in the private sector, a loss to thousands of women on the NHS.

THE COIL FAN CLUB

The fact is that most contraception for most people is a messy compromise until they find what suits them. I'm aware that telling you about the downsides of the two coils, even the temporary effects, increases reluctance in women and people assigned female at birth to try one. But better to be forewarned and forearmed with honesty than given a false picture. For most women, overall satis-faction after a year with both kinds of coils is high. Coils are the UK's most popular form of long-acting reversible contraception (LARC), followed by the implant and the injection. Women who settle down and have used the Mirena for six years have a satisfaction rate of 92 per cent, but even a follow-up survey of 100 American students who had been on the coil for just over a year showed that 83 per cent were 'happy' or 'very happy' with either kind of coil.[29] The twelve-month continuation rate was 89 per cent, and only three per cent gave up because of coil expul-sions, and six per cent had side effects. (Statistics seem to vary on this, and the copper coil is more likely to be jetti-soned by women in the first year than the hormonal one.)

Family planning services and health authorities are keen to promote the coil as cheap, safe and effective, and belt and braces in terms of pregnancy prevention as abortion rights are eroded. They also make economic sense (tell that to the NHS in the UK with its long coil-fitting waiting lists). In Colorado, back in 2008, when they removed financial barriers and improved overall access to coils, teen birth and abortion fell significantly, and the state avoided nearly $70 million in public assistance costs over five years.[30] But the satisfaction of the vast majority should not mean that we don't hear the voices of the few who have suffered (in some cases debilitating) side effects.

It seems that only around one in ten women have a long-term problem that necessitates removal – and a few just expel the coil naturally. Over 14 per cent of women use the coil worldwide,[31] and in America, where demand is growing, Planned Parenthood says coils can be free or low cost with many health insurance plans or Medicaid[32] and they may help those with low incomes. In the UK the data is limited on increasing interest in the coil, but as I met twenty-somethings doing interviews for this book, I heard more and more about women swapping from the pill to the coil. It's a hugely popular choice for women who have already had a baby, here and across Europe. In my own life, I am surrounded by coil fans, particularly medical professionals, and content long-time users. When my daughter Molly was in her final year at the University of Edinburgh, all four of her flatmates swapped from the pill to the copper or hormonal coil, but they did struggle for months to get appointments. The change has been a success for them all.

THE BEST OF COILS, THE WORST OF COILS . . .

Digging deep into the world of coils makes me think that many of the scares and temporary side effects would frighten people far less if they were honestly informed beforehand and afterwards. What if they were put in care of expert coil fitters, who had the time and skill to look at the womb and the woman holistically rather than mechanically? After all, every short-term coil-fitting cost is a long-term saving to health services in terms of future contraception, pregnancy and abortion risk. Economics alone, never mind humanity, should dictate that the process should be made more accessible and comfortable for women and non-binary and trans people who need it. We should also take the process into our own hands, choosing whether or not to change contraception, logging bleeding, cramps and symptoms afterwards on our phones or a journal, taking note of any changes in mental health. Information is power – and our own safety net. But it's not easy. As Dickens might have put it if he'd been in the sexual health business, it was the best of coils, it was the worst of coils. Now it's your choice.

CHAPTER SEVEN

ENDOMETRIOSIS, FIBROIDS AND PCOS

Hilary Mantel, the Booker Prize-winning author of *Wolf Hall*, felt the first blast of agony shortly after she had started her periods. 'As I bled, sweated and shook, something was scraping and chiselling, urgently, inside my body. I felt – and I was right – that I was leaving normal life behind.'[1]

ENDOMETRIOSIS

This was a beginning of a life plagued by endometriosis, an inflammatory condition which affects one in ten women, and which Mantel wrote about with eloquence and anger. She was gaslighted by doctors for years, diagnosed with 'stress, caused by overambition', much in the Victorian medical tradition of diagnosing overexcitement and hysteria. She was given tranquillisers and called 'Little Miss Neverwell' by one of her consultants. Mantel identified her case of endometriosis by consulting a medical textbook.

After diagnosis, she had her womb, ovaries and part of her bladder removed to get rid of endometrial tissue, rendering her infertile by the age of twenty-seven.

The damage done by endometriosis affected her until she died in 2022, but her public and honest discussion of the condition helped a huge number of women. Another high-profile case of endometriosis plagued the American filmmaker and writer Lena Dunham, who wrote about her decision – after nine surgeries – to demand a hysterectomy at the age of thirty-one to help stem her endometriosis. Her life had become unliveable with the disease. 'I try desperately to manage this new level of pain. I try so hard it becomes a second job.'[2]

These cases have catapulted endometriosis into mainstream discourse. Long ago endometriosis was described as 'the career woman's disease'. It was believed to afflict women who put off marriage and pregnancy to further their careers, a punishment for failing to bear children rather than an affliction that might cause infertility. In fact, it is endometriosis itself which disrupts women's careers. Typically, it takes seven years for white women to get diagnosed in the UK, and ten years for Black women, due to barriers to gynaecological care and systemic racism – academics cite a historic assumption that Black people had higher pain thresholds.[3]

What exactly is endometriosis?

One and a half million women in the UK live with endometriosis, and eight million in America, but unless you've got endometriosis, you've probably only the vaguest idea of what it is. The illness makes around a third of sufferers infertile, although getting pregnant often gives women a temporary respite from symptoms. People often assume endometriosis is something to do with really heavy periods, inexplicable 'women's troubles', and have no sense of the excruciating pain it can cause. The first assumption is correct: the condition can cause long, painful, tsunami-like periods. But there are often more complications, because clumps of cells similar to those in the endometrium – the womb lining – appear elsewhere in your body and leech on to other organs, making their own estrogen, and the cells' inflammation causes severe pain.[4] Endometrial cells are always shed from the lining of the uterus during menstruation, but the similar cells that are mysteriously found elsewhere in the body – in the ovaries, abdomen, bladder or even lungs – just stay put, and have no purpose apart from causing discomfort and creating hard endometriosis lesions. This can often cause painful sex and fertility problems; indeed, endometriosis is the reason for almost half of women's infertility.

These errant cells can be removed by keyhole surgery, but waiting lists are long and the endometrial tissue sometimes grows back. The earlier that endometriosis can be recognised in women and people assigned female at birth, the better, before it causes scarring and damage that can make organs stick to each other and cause adhesions that affect health and fertility. Endometriosis can cause severe pelvic pain, painful periods, pain during sex, infertility, bloating, nausea, fatigue – and that miserable package of symptoms often brings on depression, too. There's not much on offer to help with the pain, except paracetamol, ibuprofen and codeine-based painkillers. Many women just carry a hot water bottle wherever they go. While contraception can help ease the symptoms of endometriosis, it can also mask symptoms for years, making the condition harder to identify and delaying the opportunity to have early surgical intervention.

How the contraceptive pill can help with endometriosis symptoms

There is some good news, however: the combined estrogen-progestin contraceptive pill and the progestin-only pill have been shown in a number of studies to help relieve pain and inflammation in two-thirds of women with endometriosis.[5] This is because the contraceptive pill has anti-inflammatory properties and so can help to reduce the endometrial cell growth. The hormonal coil, implant and injection also have a similar effect, leaving women with a wide choice of methods. Hormonal contraception does not cure endometriosis, but often puts it on hold or lessens symptoms for a number of years.

Hormonal contraception can also reduce the recurrence of endometriosis after surgery, again by decreasing inflammation. Patients are also offered another hormonal therapy, called GnRH agonists, with names like Zoladex and Synarel, which basically block all sex hormones and send the body into temporary menopause, with all its unpleasant side effects, from mental health issues to joint pain and hot flushes. So, for some women, staying on the contraceptive pill for as long as possible is the best answer.

If women are on the pill for over a decade or more, they have to be more careful about the risk of thrombosis or clots, particularly if they are overweight or smokers, so experts suggest that women on the combined pill eventually move to the progestin-only pill as they age. As you would assume, taking the pill non-stop without a fake-bleed break helps avoid monthly flare-ups,[6] although non-menstrual pelvic pain and discomfort during sex can still occur.

On my @Pillscandal Instagram, when I asked people for good-news stories for this book about the contraceptive pill, this endometriosis experience appeared from @Pennyricketts:

'I'm so much better on the pill. Endometriosis had led me to being in bed in excruciating pain, violently sick and rocking because that's all I could do. I'd regularly feel suicidal, to the point I'd think I needed help and then, bam, I'd get my period and be like, "Oh, it's just *that* again." My acne was sorted being on the combined pill, but I had migraines with aura [headaches with flashes of light or vision changes] so I had to come off it. Then I went on to the mini pill. I'm constantly scared the anti-pill stance will change doctors' approaches. I've been taken off the pill before and have physically damaged my body due to the impact of endometriosis and not being on the pill.'

It's worth emphasising again that the pill works differently for every woman, and for some it is a godsend. We need more research on both the benefits and the risks.

How is endometriosis diagnosed?

If you suspect you have endometriosis, it is worth keeping a journal or note on your phone to chart your menstrual cycle, the heaviness of each period and any pain or symptoms, which you can then discuss with a doctor. They may offer an abdominal or vaginal examination, a pelvic ultrasound, blood tests or a scan. If they cannot diagnose anything, or those tests point to something wrong, ask for a second opinion or a referral to a gynaecologist because the gold-standard route for a definitive diagnosis of endometriosis is with a laparoscopy, an investigation done under a general anaesthetic via keyhole surgery with a tiny camera on the end of a thin, bendy tube. If the surgeon sees any patches of endometriosis, they may use laser or heat treatment to destroy them there and then, or take a tissue sample, a biopsy, to check the cells. But even when rogue endometrial tissue is removed, it sometimes grows back months or years later.

What is adenomyosis?

The same regrowth can happen with adenomyosis (an alien word my laptop's spell-checker rejects, even though it a condition also affecting 1 in 10 women), where endometrial tissue grows into the muscle in the wall of the womb. Adenomyosis was recently brought into the public eye by broadcaster and sufferer Naga Munchetty. It took thirty-five years of debilitating pain and being told to 'suck it up' before she got a diagnosis. 'I was especially told this by male doctors who have never experienced a period but also by female doctors who hadn't experienced period pain,' she said.[7] On her radio show, she revealed: 'Right now as I sit here talking to you, I am in pain. Constant, nagging pain. In my uterus. Around my pelvis. Sometimes it runs down my thighs. And I'll have some level of pain for the entire show and for the rest of the day until I go to sleep.'[8] She suffered ten-day-long periods that sometimes made her faint, and said one flare-up was so bad her husband called an ambulance after she screamed for forty-five minutes. Often adenomyosis affects women after they have children, and a hysterectomy can be a solution, but for younger women, hormonal contraception is recommended by the Faculty of Sexual and Reproductive Healthcare for relief of symptoms of adenomyosis too.[9]

Both adenomyosis and endometriosis are invisible from outside, so the start of diagnosis relies on women's experiences of severe pain being believed. Sometimes a pelvic examination will reveal the uterus has become larger or painful to touch, but an ultrasound or magnetic resonance imaging are more likely to show the changes. As Abby Norman wrote in *Harper's*: 'Doctors today often refer to the diseases that exclusively befall women – ovarian cancer, endometriosis – as "silent" and "unseen". This is unsurprising; those who are doing the describing are frequently men. Women might use different language. When you talk to the women who have had endometriosis, you will find that it isn't that the disease is silent, but that no one is listening.'[10]

Living with endometriosis

Jennifer Moore (@jen.dometriosis), a campaigner and educator from Cambridge who contacted me on Instagram, is trying to break that silence. Jennifer and I got together to discuss her endometriosis history and she recounted how awful her periods were from the start, at eleven years old, and she vividly remembers being curled up on her parents' bed, unable to stand upright. Her mother had endometriosis too, and a large UK study of DNA has shown there's often a shared genetic basis for the condition, and sensitivity to this kind of pain.'' Jennifer was put on the combined pill at the age of twelve, mostly Microgynon 30 and Logynon 20, for almost two decades to calm what doctors thought were 'just' heavy periods. It helped, but the pill breaks – the fake bleeds which we now know were unnecessary – meant that Jennifer had a 'terrible, debilitating' week every month. 'My doctor told me I just wasn't special – I was just expected to shut up and buck up every month.'

When she was thirty, Jennifer thought she would give her body a break from the pill and discovered the extent to which it had been masking her endometriosis symptoms. 'When I came off the pill, menstruation became agony; every part of my body seemed to hurt. I was crawling from my bed to the bathroom. There was blood all over me and the bathroom. I was vomiting with the pain.' She wrote everything down on a A4-side of paper and talked to her GP on the phone. 'She was quiet for a moment and then said, "I think we need to do something."' But it turned out that waiting lists for diagnosis and surgery on the NHS were at least eighteen months long, and Jennifer realised she couldn't continue living in pain. She had an MRI scan done privately, and a first round of laparoscopic or keyhole surgery to remove endometrial tissue.

When we spoke in 2023, Jennifer was recovering four weeks after a second major operation to remove endometriosis lesions and invasive tissue that was sticking her ovaries to her uterus. She looked in great health when we spoke, but the damage is inside in both senses. 'This has had a huge psychological impact. Huge. I've cried a lot. It takes away so much: your social life, your health, your intimacy, your confidence, your fertility.' The private surgeries and scans have cost around £25,000, and the constant pain meant Jennifer also had to give up her job making wedding cakes – 'those cakes are really heavy to carry' – although Chris, her partner, is supporting her in every way. 'For a couple of years, he's been my carer, and has done the housework on top of his day job. Whole families are affected by endometriosis too.

'After the first surgery, I couldn't see a version of myself without this disease. I was in a very low place. I needed outside support and therapy,' said Jennifer. What has made a huge difference has been getting involved in the 'endo' community on Instagram and campaigning and helping others. One of her posts went viral when a friend, Katherine Fletcher, who is usually a bridal make-up artist, came round and painted Jennifer's abdomen and legs with scary purple bruises and bloody red scars – showing what she was feeling inside. They posted the picture on

Halloween and added the caption: 'But you don't look sick . . . ' 'The scariest thing I could think of for this Halloween . . . what my endometriosis would look like if you could actually see how it feels and the damage it causes,' wrote Jennifer. 'I believe if more people could see this disease, they'd take it a lot more seriously.'

A new hope for diagnosis

One of the dastardly aspects of endometriosis is that the pain levels suffered do not necessarily reflect the visible extent of the disease. Some women have very little pain, and the lesions are only discovered when they have difficulty conceiving. Others, like Jennifer, find endometriosis is masked by the pill until the full extent of damage is discovered when the synthetic hormones wear off. Diagnosis takes a long time and laparoscopy, which needs to be done under general anaesthetic, is a huge expense to the cash-strapped NHS.

But there is good news about a new test for endometriosis using samples of menstrual blood.[12] Professor Christine Metz is part of the ROSE team (Research OutSmarts Endometriosis) at Feinstein Institutes for Medical Research in New York, which has been developing better ways to diagnose the condition. They have started examining period effluent gathered on a sponge on top of a normal sanitary towel. That menstrual blood contains stromal cells – the connective tissue cells of the endometrium – which turn out to be very aggressive in patients with endometriosis. The team has enrolled patients with endometriosis so it can compare menstrual results with laparoscopic test results and hopes to create a Food and Drug Administration-approved diagnostic test soon. 'In the past, in order to get to the endometrium, you would have to do a surgical biopsy and we found that you can indeed get endometrial tissue through menstrual effluent,' said Professor Metz. 'What this study is showing is that they really were able to identify differences, at a cellular, molecular level in women who have endometriosis versus women who do not.' With this window into the uterus, diagnosis could be far faster, earlier and cheaper than it is at present. The researchers expect that menstrual blood could be used to identify all sorts of other conditions from diabetes to cancer; up until now, there has been a mysterious scientific reluctance in academia to study something once considered embarrassing and disgusting.

There's one other tool in the endometriosis arsenal, and that's the use of body-identical oral micronised progesterone, a natural copy of your own hormone made from soy, rather than synthetic progestins. Some women who cannot tolerate the synthetic progestins find progesterone easier. The hormone pill goes under the name of Prometrium in the US and Utrogestan in the UK. Dr Lara Briden, author of *Period Repair Manual*, sometimes suggests it to patients with endometriosis. 'Real progesterone is gentler than a progestin, so needs to be used at a higher dose to have the same period-lightening effect.'[13] The natural progesterone has a much lower risk of clots and helps reduce the reappearance of endometrial lesions after surgery. Dr Briden also suggested that endometrial and polycystic ovarian syndrome symptoms can be helped by a change in diet;

avoiding gluten and cow's dairy among other products, as well as looking after the gut bacteria in the microbiome[14] by taking prebiotics and probiotics, and increasing consumption of a wide range of fresh vegetables and fibre.

Endometriosis sufferers are also closely watching a trial at the University of Edinburgh of a new non-hormonal drug dichloroacetate, which helps relieve endometriosis pain. Dichloroacetate is already licensed as a drug to treat rare childhood metabolic disorders and cancers, so it may be available soon. Dr Lucy Whitaker is leading the research and told the *Guardian*: 'We know women with endometriosis desperately want more treatment options and better ways to manage the often-debilitating pain that it causes. Our research so far shows promising results that dichloroacetate can make a huge difference. I hope our new trial will confirm this and give women hope that new treatments and a better quality of life are on the horizon.'[15]

FIBROIDS

There's so much going on in our uteruses that gets ignored or put in the 'Keep Calm and Carry On' bracket. But if you have really heavy periods or pain, they are warning signs, and it's worth becoming your own detective, especially where fibroids are concerned. Yes, fibroids — non-cancerous growths that develop in or around the uterus — are another crapshoot in our reproductive gear. The data from almost three quarters of a million women in the UK aged between 15–54 showed that 64 per cent had fibroids.[16] Yet hardly anyone talks about them. Most women don't know the fibroids are there unless they are serious. While they are usually symptomless, they can cause horrible flooding during periods, bloating and pain, anaemia, and sometimes grow to the size of a tennis ball or grapefruit, and need to be surgically removed.

The data also shows that Black women are more than twice as likely to get fibroids. In one small study of more than 900 women aged 25–45, fibroids were found in 36 per cent of Black patients, 22 per cent of Asian-Chinese, 13 per cent of Hispanic and 11 per cent white.[17] And generally prevalence is worse as you age. Black women also tend to get fibroids younger, which can seriously affect fertility. The American non-profit Black Women's Health Imperative explained: 'Because most Black women have fibroids at some point during their lives, the symptoms they experience might seem "normal" for them. Many girls are raised to believe painful, heavy periods are just a part of life. However, too many Black women do not have an accurate idea of what normal really is. Women suffer needlessly before seeking treatment for their fibroids . . . Black women waited substantially longer than white women before seeking treatment.'[18]

We're all waiting a long time in the UK too, since NHS England gynaecology waiting lists have gone up by 60 per cent since 2020, with over half a million women on the list, with an average delay of four months. In 2023, almost 40,000 women had waited more than a year for an appointment,[19] during which time fibroids or endometriosis grow worse. Would there be similar delays if, say, fibroids were a man's problem rather than a woman's problem? If men were growing giant fibroids on their testicles, would this area be so neglected?

I had no idea I harboured fibroids until I found I'd begun to bleed a small but regular amount on hormone replacement therapy (HRT), which included micronised progesterone, which helps thin the lining of the womb and lowers any risk of endometrial cancer. Clearly the natural progesterone wasn't protecting my womb lining from the estrogen strongly enough. Worried, I paid £95 privately for an ultrasound scan, as waiting lists post-Covid were high, and I felt I shouldn't be complaining or taking up NHS doctors' time. Despite writing two books about 'women's troubles', I was still dismissing my own symptoms and needs. It must be deeply ingrained in so many of us.

It turned out I had three small fibroids embedded in the walls of my uterus. I watched as the doctor measured them on the ultrasound scan – the biggest was three centimetres in diameter, the others over two centimetres. It looked like I had a ping-pong ball and two gobstoppers stuck to my womb – and my womb was only nine centimetres long. Estrogen makes fibroids grow, and the estrogen in HRT was growing mine and causing bleeding. I went into a panic, thinking I'd have to have a hysterectomy.

The doctor doing the scan told me to come off my HRT until I could see a gynaecologist, but I didn't want to go cold turkey. I called Dr Louise Newson, who is a friend and also runs the largest menopause clinic in the world, to get her advice. She recommended I look into the Mirena coil, as it helps thin the lining of the womb and stops the bleeding – and that is exactly what I did when I went to my NHS gynaecologist a few weeks later. I got a hormonal coil, stayed on the micronised progesterone too, which helps with mood and sleep, and I haven't had a fibroid problem or bleeding since.

How do you fight fibroids?

I was lucky as my fibroids were small, and many women find the hormonal coil or the progestin-only pill, implant or injection reduces heavy bleeding from fibroids.[20] The combined contraceptive pill can also work sometimes, as long as there is a large enough dose of progestin to counteract the estrogen. Fibroids usually shrink after menopause because the estrogen that feeds them runs out, but not if you're maintaining your natural hormones on HRT. But if contraceptive pills or coils don't help, what's the next option? Tranexamic acid tablets stop the small blood vessels in the womb lining from bleeding, so that can help, and so can endometrial ablation, surgery to thin or remove the womb lining.

Many women who tell their stories on the British Fibroid Trust website[21] (a great resource) want to keep their fertility and avoid a hysterectomy, and instead have good results with embolisation, which means blocking the blood vessels that feed the fibroid, or a myomectomy, removal of the fibroid but not the womb. A hysterectomy usually works, but it's major surgery, and about a third of hysterectomies are for fibroids. Those hormone-blocking, menopause-creating GnRH agonists are also offered to women to help shrink fibroids, sometimes before surgery, but the side effects are unpleasant. There are also good studies showing that the drug ulipristal acetate or Esmya (which is also used as a morning-after pill) helped reduce fibroid size by 42 per cent and heavy periods for 98 per cent of women. So, there are wide choices out there; be armed with information (unlike me) and ask for them.

POLYCYSTIC OVARIAN SYNDROME

Welcome to another gynaecological and psychological battleground for women and people assigned female at birth – polycystic ovarian syndrome (PCOS). Again, we find that PCOS is really common, in about 15 per cent of women aged 15–45, but how many people know exactly what it entails? 'Up to one in five women get it, yet there's no real consensus on diagnostics, solutions, and the psychological aspect gets completely ignored,' said Dr Vikram Sinai Talaulikar, an NHS gynaecologist at University College London and an expert on PCOS. He explained that some women are born with an excessive number of eggs, a large number of follicles that can cause an imbalance of hormones. Women with PCOS have extra testosterone and will not ovulate every month – periods could be every two months, six months, or not at all. They tend to get acne, on their face and body too sometimes, lose scalp hair and gain body hair and also have insulin resistance, which means it's easy to gain weight. There can also be difficulties getting pregnant. Basically, it's a feminine nightmare, a vicious, spotty circle. 'Of course, there's a spectrum – extreme for some, fine for others,' said Dr

Talaulikar. 'We find that 20 to 30 per cent of women have the worst symptoms. Others have polycystic ovaries but no syndrome, but mild symptoms.'

Aisha Torabally is thirty-two and has been a mental health worker and research co-ordinator in the NHS in Essex for years; now she's doing a Master's degree in Cultural and Global Perspectives and Mental Healthcare. She has lived with PCOS since her diagnosis ten years ago, and with her expertise, both professional and personal, is aware that PCOS affects the mind as much as the body. 'People don't talk about the mood swings that go with PCOS – half of the month I'm me, and half of the month I'm a completely different person,' she said. Dr Talaulikar has been her doctor for years, ever since she was referred up for secondary care, and they have worked together to combat the illness.

While the combined estrogen-progestin pill helps many women with PCOS, Aisha turned out to be a more compli-cated case, as she cannot tolerate the combined pill due to migraines. She tried the progestin-only Cerazette to regu-late periods, but she also has adenomyosis and fibroids with heavy bleeds, so a Mirena coil to thin her womb lining was considered as the next option. 'But that turned out to be the most horrendous thing I've ever done to myself: I had bleeding and spotting for ten months, and then I got pelvic inflammatory disease because of the coil and was hospi-talised with sepsis.' (This is rare, but the Mirena patient leaflet does warn of the risk of pelvic inflammatory disease and sepsis under possible side effects.[22]) So, it was back to the gynaecological drawing board. Aisha has tried almost all the drugs in the anti-PCOS arsenal, from tranexamic acid to reduce heavy periods, to metformin for insulin resistance and the prevention of type 2 diabetes, and spironolactone for tackling facial hair growth and acne. Because her body does not respond normally to insulin, Aisha is taking diet and exercise very seriously to keep her weight down. In an unfairly vicious cycle, insulin build-up also increases the production of androgens: 'In my thirties I'm the heaviest weight I've been at 67kg, compared to 46kg eight years ago. It does add a level of pressure,' she laughed. 'No sugar, no burgers.'

What are the best PCOS treatments?

The contraceptive pill is really helpful for the majority of women with PCOS and considered a first-line treatment. Dr Talaulikar explains that women should avoid progestin-only pills, as many of them have testosterone-like actions, and they will worsen skin problems. He advises combined estrogen and progestin pills like Dianette or Yasmin, which contain anti-androgenic progestins and a higher dose of estrogen. But the pill (as we know by now) has its own problems. 'Some women don't like the pill as it gives them an emotional crash, mood swings, and lowers libido,' according to Dr Talaulikar. 'If they've already had a lot of weight gain there's also a higher risk of blood clot.' But there are other drugs, which Dr Talaulikar tends to start if the pill isn't working well or cannot be tolerated. He offers patients metformin and spironolactone, plus Vanique to help banish chin or facial hair, or the anti-androgen tablets finasteride.

Early identification and early aggressive intervention are important in PCOS, said Dr Talaulikar. 'We really need to get our acts together. Get mothers to bring in their teenage daughters so we can help with their hormones before they put on weight. There's a higher chance of getting PCOS if it's in your family.' Aisha's mother and two sisters have PCOS, and her youngest sister has been getting help for hirsutism and acne. South Asian women have a higher tendency to PCOS, and it affects different communities differently. Dr Talaulikar, who trained in Goa, said that in India, the rate is closer to 30 per cent, and Hispanic/Latina women also have similarly high incidence.[23] Again, I'm not sure if every aspect of PCOS is a problem for everybody – I'm thinking of the handsome Mexican painter Frieda Kahlo and her delight in including the shadow of her moustache along with her monobrow in self-portraits. Not everyone has Kahlo's confidence. 'Looking in the mirror and not feeling confident is so tough. Sometimes they need counselling too. Women need to be empowered and able to get constant lifelong help when lows come,' said Dr Talaulikar.

How to manage PCOS

Dr Talaulikar is passionate about trying to increase awareness of PCOS, and the accompanying mental health side effects, among GPs and healthcare professionals. Inducing ovulation using medicines or laparoscopic or keyhole surgery on the ovaries, using heat or a laser to destroy the tissue in the ovaries that's producing androgens, such as testosterone, are also options that can help with getting pregnant. Dr Talaulikar likes to start with hormonal options, and once again, body-identical hormones look promising. He prescribes the safer body-identical hormones for women in menopause, and there are two contraceptive pills that contain body-identical estrogen, Zoely and Qlaira. Another promising option, Drovelis, is approved but not fully available yet on the NHS, and it can be bought in the US under the name Nextstellis. 'The body-identical estrogen seems to cause fewer headaches, less breast tenderness, better mood and less bloating.' Naturopath Dr Lara Briden also suggests using cyclical body-identical progesterone (Utrogestan in the UK, Prometrium in the US) in the second half of the month to help lower androgens and restore ovulation.[24]

Aisha thought it was important to explain PCOS from the patient's point of view and is happy to speak out publicly about it. 'One thing people don't factor in is pre-menstrual syndrome (PMS) and that starts at least two weeks before my period. Some women with PCOS have it worse than others, I think.' The fluctuation in her hormones triggers Aisha's heart rate, which races when she stands up from sitting or lying, and her hypermobility symptoms increase. 'My joints are more achy, or I get more drowsy. This can vary from cycle to cycle. My mood worsens too sometimes; you get triggered more easily or something that you know you can handle were you not PMS'ing feels ten times worse whilst you are PMS'ing. I'm also bigger in size because of the bloating. So I have two different sizes of clothing for pre and post period. I guess what I'm saying is having PCOS means adjusting my lifestyle month by month and being prepared for flare-ups of my other long-term conditions.' Aisha has had three years of therapy to help her cope with her chronic condition and its impact across her life. 'Therapy helps a lot. But to be honest, the only way I've coped is just by keeping going.'

It is shocking that around a quarter of women are dealing with PCOS and endometriosis, month after month, and that research has been so sluggish until now. It's taken years of effort by charities and women themselves to draw attention to these conditions, and prove the pain is achingly real. Women are only starting to understand and self-diagnose. Here, the contraceptive pill is doing useful work, far beyond its original purpose, but what more could be done with safer body-identical hormones? Big Pharma should be pouring millions into this research, but it is individuals and academics who are left to do the work. The trial of dichloroacetate for endometriosis at the University of Edinburgh has been funded by the Scottish government and the charity Wellbeing of Women. Its chief executive, Janet Lindsay, pointed out that progress was long overdue: 'It's completely unacceptable that there have been no new treatments for endometriosis in forty years.' We need to bring these previous 'silent' and 'unseen' illnesses into the light and demand better treatment.

CHAPTER EIGHT

WHAT ARE THE REAL
RISKS OF THE PILL?

Most of us dismiss the tiny print about the increased risks of blood clots, strokes and breast cancer on the leaflets in packets of contraceptive pills. That's for other people, not us, we think, chucking the leaflet in the bin. Plus, the chances of any risk are miniscule. So, we ignore the uncomfortable maths around hormonal contraception and breast cancer and instead, we feel safe amid the massive popularity and sheer normality of the pill. As for strokes and clots — those are surely the territory of our grand-parents, not us? But if 10,000 younger women take a bog-standard combined contraceptive pill like Microgynon or Rigevidon, between five and seven of them will get a blood clot within a year.[1]

STROKE — A TWENTY-FIVE-YEAR-OLD'S STORY

What if, like Holly McComish, a twenty-five-year-old theatre producer from London, you turn out to be among the five unlucky people? Holly didn't have an obvious written history of risk, but she also did not get her blood pressure measured by the doctor, as she was prescribed the combined pill over the phone after the disruption of Covid lockdown. 'The doctor did mention low mood and depression, and to stop the pill if I felt down, but nothing about the risk of clots.'

Holly was in a business meeting pitching an idea on Halloween in 2021 when she started feeling very odd. 'I picked up a glass of water and tried to have a drink, but the water fell out of the side of my mouth. I started not being able to see very clearly.' And then she found herself on the floor. Holly described it as a bizarre out-of-body experience. 'I was struggling to hear and see all these people, asking, "What's wrong?" I was thinking about what to say, but I couldn't get the words out. I was stuttering.'

Holly paused and her voice cracked. She'd told her story before, but this still felt raw. I got a lump in my throat too. She was so full of oomph and life: bouncing long brown hair, gold hoop earrings, a tight green tie-dye top and a whip-smart brain. But two years ago, she'd lain frozen on the boardroom floor. 'People were saying my name and I couldn't respond. I felt like I was paralysed.' They called an ambulance. Afterwards, she discovered that her face had dropped down on one side, a typical effect of a stroke. She also discovered that the combined contraceptive pill she had started might have caused an interruption to the blood flow to her brain.

In the ambulance, Holly came out of the paralysis, really confused as they headed for Accident and Emergency. Doctors told her she had suffered a TIA – a transient ischaemic attack or mini-stroke. They asked her if she was on oral contraception, told her to stop taking it immediately, and gave her blood-thinning medication. The hospital also referred her to the stroke rehab clinic, where she would probably be the youngest patient. 'That wasn't good news. I was embarrassed, ashamed,' said Holly. 'It felt like the worst day of my life.'

She was shaky but made a 24-hour comeback in hospital and was able to walk and talk fairly normally again. The next day she went with her mum and dad for an MRI scan, which showed detailed images of her heart and brain. Holly, who is a twin, had been born with a slight opening between the chambers of her heart; these typically close up with age. 'I never knew, because it's not dangerous on its own; it's only if you experience a blood clot.' She ended up having keyhole heart surgery, which she recovered from. But the emotional toll was heavier. 'I was afraid to go out by myself for months, thinking, "What if it happens again on the tube?"'

So how did Holly's stroke happen? What is in the combined pill that can cause blood clots in a tiny minority of women?[2] Holly was given a Rigevidon pill in August 2021, which contains levonorgestrel progestin and the synthetic estrogen ethinylestradiol – it's the recipe for the most commonly used combined pills the UK. The combination of the two synthetic hormones creates clot risk. The main risk comes from the ethinylestradiol, but adding different progestins seems to slightly increase that risk. The progestin-only pill has no clot risk, and neither does the progestin-only hormonal coil or the implant,[3] and those are better options for those with any previous conditions. In the combined pill, for some people, the synthetic estrogen is associated with inflammatory changes and negative effects on blood pressure, blood lipids and coagulation.[4] Meanwhile, the progestin increases the estrogen-associated risk of thrombosis (clots) and counteracts the estrogen's beneficial cardiometabolic effects.[5]

Holly's clot blocked the flow of blood and oxygen to the brain. Many pills in the US also contain the same ingredients, including Seasonale, Levora, Altavera, Daysee and Lessina, among others. It's worth noting that they still are among the least-risky pills for clot risk, and that a woman not using any contraception has a clot risk of 2 in 10,000 over a year anyway. But anyone who is worried about taking the combined contraceptive pill should know that the chance of clots varies between pills and goes up to between 9 and 12 per 10,000 for those who take the combined pill Yasmin, which contains a different progestin, drospirenone.[6]

It's worth knowing that all progestins are not the same for clot risk, and gestodene and desogestrel also have a similarly high rate.[7] Yet here we are giving perfectly healthy young people a drug that increases their risk of clots and strokes, because that's somehow what we put up with as women and contraceptive users. There was a major outcry about double standards during the Coronavirus pandemic, when it was reported that the Astro-Zeneca Covid-19 vaccine had a clot risk of 1 in 250,000.[8] Men and women were at risk, and some countries stopped using the vaccine. The combined contraceptive pill, with a clot risk up to 12 in 10,000, continued to be prescribed.

In the aftermath, Holly spent a lot of time alone at home, worrying and writing, thinking about how something as ordinary as contraception could nearly kill you. As a free-lancer, she didn't want to take time off work. Eventually, something started to come clear: writing comic poetry about women's cruddy experiences of health, periods and sex. This work became the slim volume *If Tits Could Talk,*[9] a wryly funny poetry collection going from masturbation to menopause to a 'Bloody Mary Shag'. Holly got funding from her university to publish the book and launched it with a stand-up poetry slam on stage at the Royal Court Theatre café in 2023.[10] Here's an excerpt, which she gave me permission to use, from the poem *What Doesn't Pill You Makes You Stronger,* which starts: 'A stroke?/ Is this a joke?/ But I'm only 25,' and ends with this advice:

> There's a common misconception
> When it comes to contraception
> Despite the vast selection
> Young women need more direction . . .
> That family histories can't be mysteries
> As they often are the clue
> To which ones will suit you best
> And which ones just aren't for you

Upon reflecting, when selecting
I should have thought about this longer
But women hear my story
And remember
What doesn't pill you makes you stronger

What are the signs of danger?

For a few weeks before her stroke, Holly was on Rigevidon, with no mood problems, but then she started to feel dizzy sometimes standing on the bus and had sudden headaches. 'I thought I'd ride it out, and that my body was just adjusting. I didn't know what to look out for.' (Here, I'm thinking we should learn from this and always listen to the warning signs our bodies are giving us.) But Holly was on one of the higher dose pills, with 30 micrograms of ethinylestradiol. Studies show those higher dose pills have a 75 per cent increased risk of stroke, compared to similar 20 microgram pills, which have a 56 per cent increased risk.[11] So aiming for a lower dose of hormones is a better option, although some women get breakthrough bleeding on lower doses. Having as much knowledge as possible of your past medical history, even as a child, is important.

Combined contraceptives – pills, vaginal rings and patches – create a tiny increase in clot risk, known as venous thromboembolism (VTE), in the arms or legs, arterial thrombosis in the heart or brain, or pulmonary embolism in the lungs, all of which can (rarely) be fatal. The risk of developing a blood clot increases for those with a history of clots, high blood pressure, high cholesterol, severe diabetes, liver disease, migraines with aura, plus smokers and women over thirty-five. There is also increased risk for women who carry the Factor V Leiden protein – an inherited gene mutation which affects blood clotting. Everyone should look out for warning signs like serious headaches, unexplained chest or leg pain or breathlessness when on the combined pill. Of course, many of the studies on clot risk were done decades ago and now increasing numbers of women who take the pill are coping with being overweight or obese, and perhaps vaping has some effect too,[12] impairing blood vessel function. The Faculty of Sexual and Reproductive Healthcare has addressed contraception and weight in guidance,[13] and women who are living with obesity (a body mass index of over 30) are advised by doctors to stop taking the combined contraceptive pill if possible and change to a progestin-only method, as they have a 12–24 times greater risk of developing a leg-vein blood clot on the combined pill.[14] Obesity causes low-grade inflammation in the body, which may make it easier for clots to form, and it also means more abdominal fat, which can slow the speed of blood flow from the legs and through the abdomen, increasing the chance of clotting. Well over half of women are overweight in the UK[15] and the US,[16] and obesity is increasing. So, too, is clot risk.

The long haul of a stroke

Holly made an amazing physical recovery from her stroke and operation, but I'm painfully aware of the psychological effect of stroke on the patient, and on family and friends around them too. My dad, Douglas Muir, smoked 40 Players Untipped a day before he moved to the gentler Silk Cut, and had a heart attack in the middle of teaching an engineering class at a Coatbridge technical college. I was out clubbing at Freshers' Week at the University of Glasgow when I got the call afterwards, and rushed back to see him. He was grey and deflated. In fact, he survived into a long retirement, but his last few years were plagued by continuing mini-strokes or TIAs like Holly's, often at night, which took a little bit of him away every time, until he couldn't walk, and then some vascular dementia began to set in.

Until I started writing this book, I somehow never imagined young people dealing with debilitating strokes like that. I was talking about it to a friend in Bristol, and she said: 'Oh, women have been dealing with this for ages. My neighbour had a stroke on the pill over forty years ago. Do you want to talk to her?'

Thus I met 77-year-old Christine Purkis, a children's author, whose stroke still affects her life to this day. She had a stroke on New Year's Eve 1980, five years after she started a high-dose combined pill called Minovlar, and long after research had been published on clot risks. In fact, the stroke came just when Christine was considering stopping the pill, aged thirty-four. 'I decided I wanted a baby, but I got a stroke instead.'

Christine had driven down to London, and was just passing Sadler's Wells Ballet when she began to feel peculiar. 'A strange headache in the back of my head grew and grew. I felt dizzy and my tongue fell out of my mouth. I was driving. I stopped and got out and sat on the pavement with the car door open until I felt all right.' Now we know TIAs should be treated urgently, as they're often a warning sign you're at risk of having a full stroke in the near future, but Christine just kept going. She went back to her brother's house in London, thinking she was too young to have anything like a stroke, and drove back to see her doctor in Bristol. 'He thought it was something to do with my spine, something that tall people got. He pushed his finger into the back of my head and I fell over. I went for an X-ray on 2 January and the world stopped spinning, but my spatial awareness was still very odd. When I drove my boyfriend around, I drove with my head out of the window looking at the curb to stay on the road.'

A few days later, at one in the morning, Christine's right arm went stiff when she reached out for a glass of water. 'My arm didn't work and I could only talk like Elvis Presley out the side of my mouth. My boyfriend called an ambulance, which couldn't find the house and came and went in the darkness. I was vomiting, but we got a taxi driver who was wonderful and agreed to drive me even though I couldn't stop being sick. In the hospital, there were lots of people running me up to ward. Then Mr Campbell the consultant appeared at my side and said: 'You've had a stroke. You're going to get better.'

Which wasn't entirely true. Christine did make an extraordinary recovery, but she had been an English teacher and never had the stamina to work full time again. Her memories of the strange days after the stroke remain: 'Everything was in double vision, and I hiccupped for two weeks, day and night. It was extraordinary.' The stroke had destroyed an area of the medulla in her brain that controlled hiccups. 'It was a very rare Lateral Medullery of Wallenberg.' I had to ask how to spell that. 'Basically, the stroke hit the bit of the brain we had when we crawled out of the swamp.' Yet another learning moment for us all. Of course, there could be some underlying condition other than the contraceptive pill that caused Christine's stroke, but the doctors felt that was the reason. 'It was completely not proven it was the pill. But I knew what it was – I never had any other problems before that.'

In recovery, Christine was fed through a tube in her nose, a bit like an imprisoned suffragette. 'I had to learn to swallow again by looking at how other people did it. When they took the tube out, everything I put in my mouth, even orange juice, felt like spikes. Friends rushed in with ice cream once I could swallow a bit. Then I had to try to sit up like a toddler all over again and learned to walk. I got out of hospital once I could stagger and went to stay with my brother.' She was sent to Charing Cross Hospital physio-therapy to learn to walk uphill again. 'They put me in with the amputees, all the men, learning to play football.' As she had been a teacher, they also tried to get Christine to teach another woman who had lost all her nouns in speech after a stroke and sent her to talk to younger patients. 'Mr Campbell said I made a fantastic recovery, but when he said that, I was so angry I threw my walking sticks down on the floor. "This is not better!" I said and marched all the way home, ricocheting from lamppost to lamppost.'

Christine's memories are so vivid, and you can still hear

in her voice what a profound effect that moment has had on her life. But she also looks at it philosophically: 'I regard myself as a guinea pig of the time. Here's the pill, this magic freedom licence to behave how you want to behave. At that stage, it was a free ticket.' Now the free ticket has been revoked, women, trans and non-binary people have to make more considered and nuanced decisions as research into the risks of the contraceptive pill advances.

BREAST CANCER

What is the increased risk on the combined pill?

Laura Price was twenty-nine and working in a high-pressure job as a financial journalist in Argentina when she found a lump in her breast. She went for a mammogram, and they said it was probably benign and advised her to return in a few months. But Laura was worried; she knew her maternal grandmother had had breast cancer in her thirties. 'I was moving to Ireland to start a job at Facebook. When I got back to Dublin, my family said I should get the lump checked out again. At first, I was reluctant to pay the 60 Euros to see a GP, but I'm so glad I did. After tests, I got the breast cancer diagnosis four months down the line, and amazingly it hadn't spread, and I was able to have surgery, chemotherapy and radiotherapy.' Throughout her treatment, friends kept saying to her, 'But you're too young to get breast cancer.' Yet lots of young women increasingly do, and experts suggest this is due to having fewer children later, and being on the contraceptive pill for longer.[17] In the UK and US, around 5 per cent of breast cancer patients are under forty years old.

Laura's surgery was a wide local excision, a bit like a lumpectomy, but it involves removing more of the surrounding tissue. She blogged about her operation and experience, particularly losing her hair and getting a wig during chemotherapy. We talked over Zoom and Laura appeared in her London living room, with her hair, which had once been long, now in a cool pixie cut. She was surrounded by colourful bookshelves, and her ginger cat Cleo slunk by. Laura said she was told to stop taking the contraceptive pill immediately upon diagnosis. 'I was on the pill from about fifteen to twenty-nine, having started it for acne initially. I had disclosed my family history of breast cancer as my maternal grandmother had had it young, so I believe I was on progesterone-only pills for most of the time, though to be honest my memory is quite hazy about it. I was on [the combined pill] Dianette for a long time too.'

Any kind of contraceptive pill is not a major cause of increased risk of breast cancer; genetics, drinking alcohol, being overweight and not exercising all increase the risk far more for the one in seven women who get the disease. (Laura was keen to stress she was a slim, marathon-running 29-year-old at diagnosis, so was simply unlucky.) The Faculty of Sexual and Reproductive Healthcare guidelines say: 'Women should be advised that current use of combined hormonal contraception is associated with a small increased risk of breast cancer which reduces with time after stopping the contraception.'[18] They say meta-analyses show an increased breast cancer risk of between

19 and 24 per cent for combined pill-users. In reality, what that means is that the risk over the next fifteen years, after using the pill for five years, was estimated at 8 extra cases per 100,000 users at age 16–20 years, and 265 extra cases per 100,000 users at age 35–39 years. Risk lowered soon after women stopped using the pill. But the figures, while low, do show that taking the pill at an early age, and coming off it after a time, is much safer than taking it when over thirty-five years old. Worth considering.

The progestin-only pill (POP) has equal risks

There was a flurry of media attention when a new observational study came out in spring 2023, looking at women in the UK primary care database.[19] They compared more than 9,000 women who had invasive breast cancer between 1996 and 2017, to more than 18,000 who did not. They combined the results with other meta-analyses and came to similar conclusions to those above: over fifteen years, a woman's increased risk of breast cancer was 8 out of 100,000 for younger women, and 265 out of 100,000 for older women. What was new was that *all* forms of hormonal contraception were included, and the progestin-only pill scored slightly higher than the combined pill on risk, as did the IUS or hormonal coil. The injection had similar risks to the combined pill. All showed a 20–30 per cent increased risk. The paper concluded: 'Given that the underlying risk of breast cancer increases with advancing age, the absolute excess risk associated with use of either type of oral contraceptive is estimated to be smaller in women who use it at younger rather than at older ages.

Such risks need be balanced against the benefits of using contraceptives during the childbearing years.'

After the survey, there were many terrifying headlines like this: 'Every type of the Pill or hormonal contraception raises risk of breast cancer by up to a THIRD, major Oxford study reveals,'[20] said the *Daily Mail*. But sexual and reproductive health groups like the FSRH started a rapid rebuttal of the horror stories; this was nothing new, just the same underlying risk that had been around for years. A Danish observational study in 2017 looking at over 11,000 breast cancer cases came to similar conclusions,[21] but people had paid less attention to that than the British study. The FSRH said: 'It is possible that use of progestogen-only [progestin] contraception does slightly increase breast cancer risk among current and recent users. However, breast cancer is relatively rare among younger women – those in the age groups most likely to be using these methods of contraception – so the 20–30 per cent increases in relative risk with progestin contraceptive use observed in this study equate to very small increases in a woman's absolute risk of developing breast cancer.'[22] And the risk fades once hormonal contraception is stopped.

I think what surprised many women was that the so-called mini-pill or POP (progestin-only pill) has as much risk as the rest. Somehow the 'mini' name sounds much safer, and it some ways it is – it can be taken when breast-feeding, and there is no increased risk of blood clots. But clearly the progestin itself is a catalyst for breast cancer in a few people, and some progestins are safer than others. For instance, dydrogesterone, which is only used in hormone replacement therapy,[23] has a much lower breast cancer risk than other progestins in HRT like norethisterone acetate or medroxyprogesterone acetate. The progestin-only pill is the most popular method of contraception in the UK. Like most contraceptive pills, it is available free in pharmacies, and in the US, the Food and Drug Administration has approved Opill, a progestin-only pill, to be sold over the counter in 2024. Even though more is known about the slight increased breast cancer risk, women are left to consider this for themselves, rather than being asked about their history by their primary care doctors. But there's a trade-off with freedom to get the pill, particularly for those who live in families and communities where there's still stigma around contraception, and a question of convenience too, for the many women who do not have time to get a doctor's appointment for their next prescription.

Do different progestins in the pill have different breast cancer risks?

Dianette, which Laura used for a time, is a combined pill with 35 micrograms of ethinylestradiol synthetic estrogen, one of the higher dose pills with increased risk. (The Dianette patient leaflet notes there is a tiny increased risk of breast cancer but it is rare among women under thirty-five.[24]) But the progestin in Dianette is cyproterone acetate, which in one mouse breast tissue study[25] seemed to be one of the safer progestins for breast cancer risk, along with the progestin drospirenone. Mice mammary glands are pretty much all we have to go on, due to research costs. Some big observational studies on different progestins and breast cancer risk show completely variable results.[26] No one is racing to fund this sort of research, least of all pharmaceutical companies. (Some work has been done by academics on the progestins in hormone replacement therapy,[27] though, and basically the synthetic progestins get the thumbs down for breast cancer risk; micronised progesterone, which is extracted from soy and a copy of the human hormone, is much safer. But that's not available as contraception.)

Besides, like many women, Laura has been on a bunch of different pills and with different progestins over fourteen years, so it's hard to draw any conclusions, and there's no way to prove any connection at all between the pill and cancer, particularly as Laura found out afterwards that she had inherited a genetic mutation called PALB2. 'It's essentially like BRCA, and means I was born with something like a 50 per cent chance of getting breast cancer in my lifetime, so it's possible if I'd known that, I might not have taken the pill, but at the same time the pill helped with other issues like acne and migraines.' Laura's cancer is both estrogen-and-progesterone-receptor positive, which means both the hormones (synthetic or natural) could stimulate the growth of the cancer, so it is possible that the pill was one of the many contributing factors to her diagnosis. No one really knows.

Breast cancer risk for nuns, daughters and sisters

Family history does matter, but so do life circumstances. In fact, the group which has the some of the highest rates of cancer in later life is Catholic nuns.[28] The life of chastity means they lose out on the breast cancer-protective effects of pregnancy and breastfeeding, and the contraceptive pill decreases the risk of ovarian and womb cancer by 30–50 per cent.[29] So there are pros and cons to the combined or progestin-only pill. If you have no risk of breast cancer in your family, but an inherited risk of ovarian or womb cancer, then the pill looks like a useful protective option. On the other hand, if your mother or sister has had breast cancer, you may want to avoid the pill and the hormonal coil, even though the risk is small, and smaller still with the newer lower-dose pills. I dug into research, done in 2000, into thousands of relatives of breast cancer patients who had been treated at the University of Minnesota Hospital.[30] It showed that sisters and daughters of the patients taking oral contraceptives had triple the normal breast cancer risk; more so if they carried a mutation in the BRCA1 or 2 gene, which increases the chances of breast and ovarian cancer. But granddaughters and nieces did *not* have an elevated risk. A big caveat here is that many of the patients had been on much higher-dose pills from the 1970s that are no longer used.

What's the breast cancer risk for Black and Asian women?

As ever, when we look at cancer rates, the research is so often white-dominated, and the risks for other communities and groups is not always explained. For instance, when young Black women get breast cancer in the US, they have double the mortality rate of young white women, which is appalling, and makes knowledge around the safest contraception choices doubly important. Black women are disproportionately affected by more aggressive cancers, like triple-negative breast cancer, but structural racism and economics play their part as well. One American study worked out that 37 per cent of Black women's excess mortality risk could be explained by a lack of private health insurance, and the types of tumour only affected cases by 23 per cent.[31] Internationally, Asian women have a slightly lower rate of breast cancer than white women, but it obviously varies by country.[32] In Britain, Black women are more likely to have breast or ovarian cancer diagnosed later.[33] Health inequalities remain massive, and need to be challenged.

Even pictures of cancer patients seem so often to be white, and Black Women Rising, which supports women of colour with cancer in the UK, recently curated an exhibition of portraits showing the reality and telling women's stories. 'I think there was a feeling of freedom, of being heard,' said the charity's founder Leanne Pero (now an MBE). Leanne is a dance teacher in London who started her first Black Women Rising support group after her own bout with breast cancer: 'I thought, why don't we all come together? I got my mum to bake loads of cakes. We took kettles and cups down there and there wasn't a dry eye in the house. These are women who have not had a space to express themselves,' she said in a video.[34] Since then, the charity has gone on to provide vital help, information and practical advice for people of colour who have been diagnosed with cancer, and also tries to overturn 'the taboos surrounding cancer within the community which stopped people from speaking out about their ordeals'. Lack of awareness can lead to the devastating late-stage diagnoses and higher mortality rates in Black cancer patients compared to their white counterparts.

WHEN IT'S TIME TO COME OFF THE PILL

Many of us start the contraceptive pill as teens taken by our mothers to the doctor to sort out embarrassingly heavy bleeding or soul-destroying acne. Charlie Gowans-Eglington, a 35-year-old fashion and lifestyle journalist living in London, went on the pill aged thirteen after other treatments for her acne had failed, and stayed on it until she was almost thirty. She came off the pill overnight after seventeen years, the day she discovered her sister had been diagnosed with breast cancer, aged thirty-two. 'It was a snap decision . . . It had been at the back of my mind that the pill might be putting me at risk, but doctors had always told me not to worry, that any risk was too low to worry about.'[35] This was despite the fact that both her grandmothers and an aunt had died of breast cancer. Charlie tried various pills, but spent a decade on Dianette, with its higher dose of synthetic estrogen.

In an article in *The Times*, Charlie explained that after doctors discovered her sister's BRCA2 gene, she was tested too. 'The odds are one in two for every child of someone with BRCA. I won the coin toss, making my risk as low as the next person's.' But her mother found cancer in her breast eighteen months after Charlie's sister was diagnosed. 'Mum took the contraceptive pill for at least a decade,' Charlie wrote, although research shows the risk goes down to normal after a number of years. Charlie said she was staying away from hormonal contraception, while many of her friends remained on it, and believed there needs to be another option. 'I'm used to paying a higher price than men for my sexual freedom; the physical cost of living life as I choose to. But these risks are too high. I sat with my sister through chemotherapy, and I sat with my mum through radiotherapy. A rise in breast cancer risk is not an acceptable risk. And a double mastectomy isn't an acceptable pound of flesh.'

LOOKING FOR ANSWERS

For many cancer survivors, guessing what caused the disease (and what might cause it to recur) is an impossible itch that needs to be scratched. We know that being over-weight, drinking heavily and eating lots of ultra-processed foods increases the risk of cancer,[36] but Laura Price was a slim marathon runner and a healthy eater at the time of her diagnosis, so thinks she was simply unlucky. She looked at other areas too: 'If I'd had a pregnancy in my late twenties, like my mum, I might not have had breast cancer.' We know that hormone-receptor positive breast cancer risk decreases the earlier you have a baby, and the longer you breastfeed.[37] Laura was not offered a chance to freeze her eggs before chemotherapy and radiotherapy put her into early menopause. 'I didn't have time to stimulate my ovaries and harvest eggs before that. It feels like a slap in the face that I'm not able to have children.'

The psychological effects are often as hard as the

physical ones. Laura also wonders about carrying the PALB2 gene mutation and the catalyst of stress, particularly in her twenties. 'Stress lowers the immune system. I had a really stressful job in my twenties, writing financial news at speed with four screens open in front of me, sometimes in Portuguese too, and I had to get up at 4.45am to be at my desk for 6am, and I was staying up late with my flatmates. A burst of stress is good for you, but constant stress is bad.' There are no definitive answers, just questions, but for anyone thinking of going on the pill who has a close family history of breast cancer, I think it's worth discussing them. It's also worth knowing some good news: women who exercise for just twenty minutes a day lower their risk of recurrence of breast cancer by 55 per cent.[38]

SINGLE BALD FEMALE (30) SEEKS . . .

Laura made a good recovery after her cancer and went on the estrogen-suppressing drug tamoxifen for nearly ten years, while rebooting her career. 'I was travelling the world as a food writer, and doing a podcast, but I was also dealing with hot flushes and aches and pains, perimenopausal symptoms.' She also started internet dating and decided to be honest in her profile about cancer and losing her hair. This was chronicled amusingly in an article in the Huffington Post 'Single, Bald Female (30) Seeks . . . '.[39] To her surprise, she got some amazing replies. 'In the end, I decided I didn't want to meet someone who would turn around when I told them I'd had breast cancer and might not be able to have kids and say, "I don't want be with you."' The article went viral. 'I think the honesty resonated with a lot of people, not just the ones who'd had cancer, but people with other disabilities or mental health problems, which are not barriers, but reasons to love them.'

Thanks to her journalism, Laura, who is now thirty-nine, gets contacted by many younger women coping with cancer, asking about everything from her treatment to whether wearing a cold cap during chemo prevents hair loss, and 'scanxiety': feeling anxious about scans. She tells them to speak up around fertility and egg freezing, which is now much more common than it was when she was diagnosed. 'I was unable to freeze my eggs, and I was also single at the time.' That situation was particularly hard in her thirties, when all her friends were getting married and having children. Now Laura lives with her husband, who has three children. (He was bringing in the Sainsbury's order behind the scenes while we were on Zoom.) Laura advises younger women to advocate for their own health. 'If you feel something is wrong with you, don't be afraid to ask for a second opinion, ask for more options, be proactive, think about your future life too. Is there therapy available to you? Don't be afraid to ask, and write everything down.' Good words of advice, not just for women with cancer, but anyone looking after their menstrual, sexual and mental health.

Having been cancer-free for ten years, in 2022 Laura started getting pains in her chest, on her sternum bone, and once again it took months for this to be diagnosed. It turned out to be secondary cancer. She was devastated, and underwent major surgery to remove her sternum and the cancerous cells. The bone was recreated with 'surgical cement', she explained, showing me a thin pinkish scar on her upper chest. 'Hopefully that will stop it recurring. You can live with secondary breast cancer for a long time.' She has also been given the estrogen-blocking drug letrozole and zoladex, which puts women into chemical menopause to stop hormones.

Most people would be on their knees at this point, but Laura seems astonishingly positive and unstoppable, and took her experience by the scruff of the neck by writing *Single Bald Female*, a novel which came out in 2022,[40] before her secondary breast cancer diagnosis a few months later. The book is funny, devastatingly honest, and has been hugely reassuring for thousands of readers. Ever resilient, Laura got rejected by a few publishers until a major one, Macmillan, picked up her book. 'It is so good to walk into a bookshop, and see the yellow cover and the girl with the blue wig,' she said.

So that's the real story behind the statistics, the possible increased risk of clots and breast cancer on the pill, told by three writers: a poet, a children's book author and a novelist. They are searingly articulate about what's happened, what it's like to be the one-in-a-thousand case, the unlucky one, and they have turned their misery into a creative metamorphosis. Apart from admiring their resilience, what else we can learn from all this?

For starters, it would help if we were all better informed about the warning signs of a stroke or clot, and if more women with cancer in the family were able to have early genetic testing, so they could make informed decisions. We also need to be better informed about what's in whichever pill we're taking so we can make a safer choice. We know a high dose of synthetic estrogen is riskier for breast cancer, and certain progestins are riskier for clots. As I mentioned in Chapter 1, there are newer combined pills available made with body-identical estrogens: Zoely and Qlaira with estradiol, and Drovelis (or Nextstellis in the US) with estetrol. The body-identical estrogens seem to have a much lower clot risk in trials so far[41] – Zoely is estimated at 2 cases per 10,000 women per year and Drovelis is estimated at 3.6 – both pretty close to the normal level of risk without hormonal contraception.

But these pills are more expensive, so your healthcare provider may be reluctant to prescribe them. In the UK, Drovelis costs around £8 a month, compared to older pills which cost just under £2. Aren't we worth that? Apparently not. The NHS barely prescribes Drovelis, so women are buying it privately, but you can get Zoely and Qlaira in some areas. Moving out to the bigger picture, why has it taken so long for there to be a better-tolerated pill, and why were we allowed to tolerate strokes and clots for sixty years, as a side effect? Why should we be compromising like this still? Why should we have to put up with this collateral damage around our contraception?

CHAPTER NINE

DO DIGITAL CONTRACEPTION APPS REALLY WORK?

In what may be an international first, interviews with two of the women in this chapter were both conducted while they were breastfeeding their new babies, on the phone, and looking after a toddler at the same time. Plus, they both made sense. But while yoga teacher Tessa Clemson got pregnant intentionally, the other, Labour councillor Kate Walsh, was carefully using the Natural Cycles app and measuring her temperature every day for fertility awareness contraception when she conceived. Kate is thirty-three and has been going to Tessa's preganacy and mother and baby yoga classes in Great Harwood, Lancashire, for a couple of years, where the conversation around hormone-free birth control and 'green sex' is growing, as it is worldwide, from Instagram and TikTok to books and classes. Indeed, we filmed part of the *Pill Revolution* documentary at Tessa's studio – and five new mums turned up who had accidentally got pregnant while using fertility awareness methods. Oops.

FEMTECH AND THE FRUITION OF FERTILITY AWARENESS

I think the increasing knowledge of synthetic hormones and the effects they have, particularly on mental health, is bringing femtech and the fertility awareness movement to massive fruition. Women want to understand and be in sync with their cycles. Digital period apps like Flo, Clue, and fertility awareness apps like Natural Cycles are used by hundreds of millions of women round the world. Constant intimacy with our phones — which are also sometimes our friends and confidantes — has brought us new intimacy and insight into our menstrual cycles, and a deeper understanding of how hormones rollercoaster through our moods throughout the month. Apps are sometimes like having an ancient wise woman to consult in your pocket. Particularly for younger women and trans men and non-binary people, these apps can be hugely reassuring and a safe space to ask awkward questions. However, there remain some doubts around femtech. Which apps are still harvesting our health data for their own profit? And are the claims of effectiveness on fertility apps true? For instance, Natural Cycles says it has a 'typical use effectiveness rate of 93 per cent and a perfect use effectiveness of 98 per cent'.[1] So that's a 7 per cent fail rate in the real world, compared to a 1 per cent failure rate on the hormonal coil. Kate is part of that 7 per cent failure rate and had her second baby a lot closer to her first child than she intended, after putting her trust in Natural Cycles. 'I went on it when my first baby was eighteen months old, and I got pregnant within three months of using the app, and I didn't even know I was pregnant again until five or six weeks because everything looked normal.'

'Don't forget to abstain on a red day!'

Kate was very careful to measure her basal body temperature (a reading taken when you are fully at rest) at the same time every day upon waking, and entered that and her period dates into the app. She had sex with her husband on days her phone showed her a green circle with the words 'Not Fertile' on it and abstained on the red circle 'Use Protection' days. The Natural Cycles app provides a calendar with green and red days, and periods are indicated with a green circle with a drip in it. 'The algorithm will use your temperature to calculate your fertility status for the day. "Don't forget to use protection or abstain on a red day!"' it says, advising people to use male or female condoms. When I set up the app myself just to experiment, I found that ten days of each month were red, with the green safe days appearing during your period and at the start of the first follicular stage of the cycle. Then you are likely to be fertile in the days before ovulation, and for a few days after into the later luteal phase that leads up to your next period. Your temperature starts to go up minutely as ovulation approaches – from roughly 36 to 37 degrees Celsius – and you can also narrow that window by measuring any surge in luteinising hormone (LH), which means your body is trying to start ovulation. The app suggests when you should test for this, and sells LH strips to pee on a couple of times a month, which look a bit like mini pregnancy tests, at £18 for fifteen. The 'Gen 2 thermometer' costs £29.99, but this is included in the basic subscription to the app at £69.99 a year. When Kate used the app a few years ago after her first child, the extra LH test was not in existence, so it was perhaps slightly less accurate.

'I fell pregnant after three months on Natural Cycles'

'I was eighteen when I first went on the mini-pill [progestin-only] and I had issues with weight gain on it, tried to find a better one, and then came off it just before I got married. In fact, I was pregnant by the time I got married,' Kate said, laughing. 'I went back on the pill after my first child, and it just never settled. I was bleeding every fourteen days, and the doctors said: "You've just got to persevere."' Kate had been made redundant from her debt-rewriting job a few months before – she had received the message while she was in labour in hospital. (Maternity leave is not popular with some employers, and she was told she had to apply for another role within seven days.) Instead, she decided to study history and politics at university, which was life-changing, but after a year she was still bleeding constantly on the mini-pill and said: 'I didn't really have time to go to the doctors – I only go if I'm really sick or pregnant or something, and the nurse I saw said she couldn't change my pill – only the doctor could.' She used to go to the local Brook sexual health services clinic, but that service stops when you are twenty-five years old. Frustrated, Kate was on Facebook when she saw an advert for Natural Cycles. 'I was just desperate, and I thought I'll give it a go. For three months it was fantastic. My mental health improved massively not being on the pill. I'd felt rubbish after having the baby.' Then she fell pregnant. 'I thought, no way can I be pregnant on this app. The only way I could be pregnant is if I'd ovulated a week early.' Which was obviously what had happened – Kate's short cycle pattern and lower body temperature didn't mesh with the algorithm of the app. 'I told them what happened, but they never contacted me.' Of course, Natural Cycles cannot guarantee their fertility tracking will work for everyone, and there's this legal disclaimer on their website: 'We are passionate about empowering You with knowledge. However, it is important to note that information provided by us should never be considered medical advice.' They add, 'You understand that the accuracy of the information provided by the Services may depend on individual circumstances which cannot be known or foreseen by Natural Cycles.'² So Kate and her husband welcomed the too-early baby in the end, and a few years later they had their third child, Nancy, who was nine days old when we spoke and made contented slurping noises down the phone. It's a delightful sound, enough to make anyone throw their contraception in the bin.

The 'Hungover' button

But it does help if babies arrive in the right time and place, and Natural Cycles explain that there's more to do than just using a thermometer every day. The temperature changes can be affected by other variables, and there are three little symbol buttons for sickness, sleep disruption and hangovers, all of which can alter your temperature reading, and it is then discounted. 'Your basal body temperature can be affected by alcohol. A glass of wine or two over dinner will likely not affect your temperature, but if you drink more and wake up feeling hungover, you should choose "Hungover" to exclude your temperature,' advises the app. A fever, jet lag or sleep disruption of more than two hours can make a difference too, and they suggest you wake up to take your temperature at the weekend, and then have a lie-in. Really? Recreational drugs can seriously mess with your internal heating too, which might show up as an ovulation-like high temperature, but the app doesn't offer a 'Stoned' button. Clearly a lot can go wrong if you either have irregular cycles, or a wild, unpredictable life. Using Natural Cycles as contraception takes some dedication.

Influencers go hormone free

But go on TikTok or Instagram and there is a massive positive spin on fertility apps and a negative take on hormonal contraception. Celebrities and influencers say they have been on Natural Cycles for years and give the impression that fertility awareness is as easy as getting a fake orange tan. There's a hilarious series of influencer posts from 2021[3] plugging Natural Cycles, and various reality TV stars including Jessika Power, Lucy Mecklenburgh and Olivia Attwood Dack (who have about 4 million followers between them on Instagram) speak out from their beds or sofas while perfectly coiffed and fully dressed, waving the pink thermometer. All of them use many of the same unlikely lines: 'It's 93 per cent effective with typical use and 98 per cent effective with perfect use,' and it's 'the first FDA-cleared and only CE-marked contraceptive' and 'It's 100 per cent hormone free!' Someone should have written more convincingly colloquial scripts for them. They aren't taking their temperatures late and hungover after a night on the tiles, obviously. Other fans just say simply: 'A year ago Natural Cycles changed my life. This is my one year off birth control "happy dance".' I think it does change many people's lives, especially if they have predictable, regular cycles and discipline about using condoms. It's the most popular method of contraception on The Lowdown Review site.

In the mysterious way that the spyware on our phones listens to us and provides ads to suit, Kate found that quite soon after she discussed going back on contraception with her midwife after birth, her TikTok suddenly lit up with posts mentioning Natural Cycles. 'It seemed like almost aggressive advertising. Women saying how amazing it was to come off the pill and how well fertility apps were working for them.' She signed up to Natural Cycles, and she now believes that 'people need to be warned it's not as simple or perfect as it seems on Twitter or TikTok'. Kate put up her own @northwestkate post, talking about all the women saying their skin or bodies had improved since they came off the pill. 'This is what happened to my body when I came off the pill . . . ' she says and turns to the camera to reveal she is heavily pregnant. From the beginning, there has been an attempt at regulating the truth. In 2018, the Advertising Standards Authority in the

UK said a Natural Cycles advert had been misleading and breached the code by claiming it was a 'highly accurate contraceptive app' and a 'clinically tested alternative to birth control methods'.[4] Kate's complicated experience of contraception, fertility and maternity were some of the catalysts that pushed her to stand for her local Hyndburn Borough Council. 'There aren't many young women on the council, and I'm bringing up more motions on women's health.'

The Apple watch is watching you

Natural Cycles was the first app to link up with the Oura Ring, which costs about £200 and can measure your finger temperature and send it direct to your phone every morning when you wake up. I got a press release in autumn 2023 which announced: 'Natural Cycles has received clearance from the US Food and Drug Administration (FDA) for its Apple Watch integration. The integration will allow the Natural Cycles app, an FDA Cleared Class II medical device in the US to sync wrist temperature data from users who wear an Apple Watch with temperature-sensing capabilities overnight.' At this point, fertility apps have almost become integrated into our bodies. The Natural Cycles CEO, Dr Elina Berglund Scherwitzl, added: 'At a time when birth control accessibility has never been more important, we're excited to give millions of women who already own an Apple Watch access to deeper fertility insights.' After a google, I was also excited to know that Dr Scherwitzl was part of the team that discovered the Higgs boson particle with the Large Hadron Collider at

CERN, which led to the Nobel Prize in Physics in 2013 before she co-founded Natural Cycles. So these fertility apps are indeed smart, and let's face it, they will probably be of more importance to mankind and womankind than the Higgs boson. If only we spent that sort of money on contraceptive research . . .

GREEN SEX

There is definitely a tipping point happening around fertility and menstrual awareness. Tessa Clemson teaches dozens of women of all ages every week in her yoga studio, and she said that the conversation questioning hormonal contraception and going natural is huge. 'Everyone thinks the premise is good if you fully understand how these apps work, but I've had lots of mums coming off the pill, going on an app, saying they want to get pregnant in six or twelve months, and getting pregnant straightaway. Some of them are just super fertile.' Tessa also pointed out that women feel comfortable being honest about it all with other mums in the studio, 'whereas outside someone might be having IVF or a miscarriage, and it's sensitive.' She says the apps have also been helpful for women struggling to have a baby, 'although I tell them that they shouldn't just have sex when it says "fertile green day" – they should go for it.' Tessa is thirty and started the pill at eighteen – 'we thought there was only Microgynon back then' – then abandoned hormonal contraception for ever when she came off the pill to try for a baby. 'I felt like a cloud had lifted. I had no idea.' She and her partner Lucas now use condoms, and she also tracked her cycle on the Flo app (which doesn't measure temperature). 'It was useful — I'd be all grumpy with him and he'd ask, "Um, what bit are you at on your app?" It made me feel in control.' Lucas and Tessa now have two children, Frances and baby Bobby, who snacked away contentedly as we spoke. 'When you understand your own hormones, you have much more faith in yourself,' said Tessa. 'My partner and I have had really healing conversations now we both understand what's going on.'

Catholics and the Rhythm Method

Tessa said the older menopausal women coming to yoga were not surprised by the upsurge of interest in fertility awareness apps, and they said: 'We just called that the Rhythm Method. It's not much different.' Flo and Clue offer fertility tracking without taking temperatures, which can be used as a somewhat unreliable sort of contraception, more like the calendar-based Rhythm Method, the only form of contraception approved by the Catholic Church in 1951. As the satirist and writer H. L. Mencken pointed out at the time: 'It is now quite lawful for a Catholic woman to avoid pregnancy by a resort to mathematics, though she is still forbidden to resort to physics or chemistry.'

But what if we bring in a little more chemistry? Another useful signal of fertility can be changes in cervical mucus, explained Sarah Panzetta, who is a fertility awareness practitioner at Fertility UK[5] which is linked to the NHS website. The NHS claims natural family planning, can be 'up to 99% effective when used consistently and correctly'.[6] Sarah explained that around ovulation the mucus becomes 'a gloopy fluid, like raw egg white'. Add that detective work to your temperature, and you will improve your chances of using fertility awareness effectively. She also said luteinising hormone (LH) tests can be helpful, if pernickety, and that some of her clients use the old-school version of LH tests – cervix checks – alongside temperature.   The cervix tends to be harder when infertile, but higher and softer around ovulation. 'Lots of younger women who have been on the pill for years find connecting with how their cycle works reassuring and empowering.' Sarah specialises in helping women take back control of their cycle and work out the best fertility window for getting pregnant. 'Apps like Natural Cycles are making a lot of money out of something you can do by yourself.' Tracking cycles is reassuring and empowering for women – and men. 'Men get such an easy ride on contraception, and all we're asking them to do once you have the fertility method working is to use condoms two or three days a month.' It's also worth remembering, folks, that the withdrawal method has a 22 per cent failure rate.

'Your app knows you got your period. Guess who it told?'

There was a telling mention in the Natural Cycles' press release of the importance of cybersecurity, especially within women's health. What's happening to all the data of hundreds of millions of women on period and fertility apps? Is it being harvested like fertile eggs? Is it being used to improve academic knowledge of women's health? Is it safe? Certainly, there is more regulation in this area since the Flo Period & Ovulation Tracker app, which has over 100 million users, was taken to task in 2021 by the American Federal Trade Commission for sharing sensitive health data with marketing and analytics firms, including Facebook and Google,[7] resulting in a great headline in the *New York Times*: 'Your app knows you got your period. Guess who it told?'[8] No one knows quite how the data was used. Were giant bars of chocolate and weepy rom-coms marketed to women who were having a pre-menstrual binge? Now Flo and other apps must receive your consent to data use. I signed on as a younger version of myself, and Flo said: 'Nice to meet you Kate! Allow Flo to track your activity across other companies' apps and websites?' They also wanted me to tick the box: 'I agree that Flo may use my personal data (except health data) to send me product or service offerings via email or the Flo app.' They also asked me for access to all the health data on my phone, like the number of steps I walked each day. I said no. But we share intimate data with apps that we would only share with a doctor, who would be bound by a strict patient privacy law. The UK watchdog Privacy International discovered as far back as 2018 that a number of other menstrual apps were sharing data too.[9]

'Tap and hold the Flo logo to commit'

Yet aside from the harvesting of data, there is much to be learned from using one of these period apps, and one in five women of fertile age in the UK and US have downloaded them. Just being in tune with your cycle and its levels of grumpiness, creativity and horniness throughout the month is useful, and it's always better to blame our hormones rather than ourselves. The Flo app has more than 100 million users worldwide and seems to be aimed at a younger and less sophisticated demographic than the fertility awareness apps. As one user, Stargirl Michaela, says, endorsing Flo, 'I understand my body so much more now thanks to Flo, truly a game changer!' Meanwhile user Hymmyo adds, 'The most accurate ever! I can't believe how accurate this app is!! It almost knows to the minute honestly.' Flo offers medical advice, with sections on how to spot polycystic ovarian syndrome and endometriosis, and a chance to log your symptoms daily – mood swings, spotting, tender breasts, bloating, headaches, discharge, backache, cramps. Flo says, 'It's totally normal to feel a bit uncomfortable talking about periods. You can ask anonymous questions to the Flo community and get insights you can trust from medical experts. In fact, one in two users say Flo helps them be more open about their symptoms and how they make them feel.' There are also more fun articles, such as 'Do you want to change anything about your sex life?' or 'Make masturbation work for me'. Plus, there is a video course: 'Mastering Your Orgasm'. (Shouldn't that be 'Mistressing'?) After that tour, many women will be keen to sign up. Another page appeared: 'I, Kate, will use Flo to improve my relationship with my period, know my body better and be ready for anything. Tap and hold the

Flo logo to commit.' I committed. Flo wanted £29.49 for a year's subscription. I said no. It then made me a '33% off forever' offer at £19.99 a year. Just a tip there if you're signing up.

Menstrual tracking

I got 23-year-old English graduate Katie Scott to sign up to the Clue app and tell me what she thought. Clue is mostly for period tracking, but also offers a 'Conceive', 'Pregnancy' and 'Perimenopause' option. (That's rather useful, as periods go bonkers in perimenopausal women, usually in their forties, with erratic cycles. Plus about half of women get extra-heavy periods.) Katie, who did GCSE biology, said: 'We were taught virtually nothing about this at school. It's so bad we know so little about our bodies and cycles.' For instance, using the app she realised the first day of her period was 'Day 1' and not the day after her period finished. 'They explained the menstrual cycle and ovulation in biology, but there was no explanation of how it affects mood and energy.' Shouldn't being able to track and understand your cycle every month be the most basic part of what we teach girls – and boys – in school? Katie and I looked through Clue and she could enter data covering changes in feelings, energy, food cravings, social life, sex life, discharge, weight gain, skin, hair in the free version of the app, but she would have to sign up to the flat £7.99 fee for the first year (£5.99 a month after that) to enter data on sleep quality and breast changes. Katie would also have to pay to access many of the (well-written and footnoted) articles giving medical and contraceptive method information. We had a little trawl round the pregnancy section too, and there you could enter data on your 'Pregnancy Superpowers' including super smell, super taste, more intense orgasms and pregnancy glow. All very cheery.

I interviewed Clue's former medical director, American obstetrician, gynaecologist and reproductive endocrinologist Dr Lynae Brayboy. (Since our talk she has moved on to become an independent fertility specialist in London.) We began by discussing how prehistoric bones had been dug up by archaeologists with twenty-eight marking lines on them. Probably not man's first attempt at a calendar, but woman's first attempt at creating a menstrual app, so to speak. 'It's so useful for women to know what's normal for them, what's the baseline, and then they know when something is off,' said Dr Brayboy. 'Things like pre-menstrual migraines start making sense to women, and they can take action.' She also hoped that work she helped oversee at Clue will advance medical research, which has been criminally neglected. 'Getting funding for women's reproductive health research is very hard, and we need so much more work, particularly on non-hormonal contraception, new methods and conditions like endometriosis. There's a lot we don't know about oral contraceptive pills – some individuals need them for acne and self-esteem, and hormonal contraception can be very effective.' Different contraceptive choices are examined in detail on Clue. 'We have been giving everybody the same thing, much the same pill, and women need to know how to personalise that more,' said Dr Brayboy.

Clue is based in Germany, and there are tighter data

laws in the European Union. 'When you track in Clue, your de-identified data becomes something powerful: data that can help answer questions to better understand menstrual and reproductive health, and ultimately, to improve healthcare,' says the website,[10] adding that Clue does not sell data. They say they only share anonymous data that is relevant to the specific research, and make sure it cannot be traced back to any individual. There are some impressive projects being financed, including the Covid pandemic's impact menstrual cycles; how different people experience 'heavy menstrual bleeding', in partnership with the Bill and Melinda Gates Foundation, and how sleep and stress impact teens' menstrual cycles, with the University of California in Berkeley. Dr Brayboy was pleased that Clue was committed to diversity too. As a Black woman she believes that 'The real thing with science is it's actually not a very diverse place, but Clue's team are a diverse science team, not only in terms of training but also racially, and in thought processes, and background, and origin.'

Clue's *Hormonal* podcast tackles the science behind hormones and contraceptive access in the wider culture and tries to be LGBTQI+ inclusive: 'We know lots of women who have periods and lots who don't. We also know that people who aren't women have periods too and we also know we have listeners who have never had periods,' said the introduction. You've got to applaud the attempt to help everyone be better informed – and to advocate for themselves. Dr Brayboy mentioned Black poet and writer Audre Lorde's essay *The Cancer Journals* (which I quote at the front of this book) in which she discussed, philosophically and personally, her breast cancer and mastectomy. The words which stood out for Dr Brayboy were these: 'Every woman has a militant responsibility to involve herself actively in her own health.' I strongly agree with that.

CHAPTER TEN

TRANS AND NON-BINARY CONTRACEPTION

'I am in pain. It isn't normal. Please listen.'

Those were the words 24-year-old Dee Whitnell used to describe their frustrating personal experience around contraception and sexual healthcare. Dee identifies as non-binary and is deeply involved in the needs of the trans community in this area. They work as a sex educator and activist, write for *PinkNews* and recently completed an MA in Gender, Sexuality and Culture at Birkbeck University in London. Their @s3xtheorywithdee Instagram account charts a fluid journey of self-discovery, and provides advice alongside humour. They have spoken out against being misgendered and deadnamed (the use of their birth name after their name has been changed) by healthcare professionals. Yet, when Dee suffered excruciating pelvic cramps and made a panicked visit to A&E, they said: 'I had to put my identity aside to get the help I needed: pain first, pronouns after.'

Since then, Dee has officially changed their name and records, but for many trans people medical visits are queasily triggering in terms of gender dysphoria – the sense of discomfort someone has because of a mismatch they feel between their biological sex and their gender. Ever since Dee came off the combined contraceptive pill in their early twenties due to the constant headaches, they have struggled with intense periods and chronic pain. An ultrasound didn't show any problems, 'but further testing found polycystic polyps on my ovaries, my ovaries are enlarged, but they won't diagnose me. I don't feel I'm being listened to.' Of course, we know from previous chapters that diagnosis of the mysteries of endometriosis, adenomyosis or polycystic ovarian syndrome can take years for the average cis woman, but there's an added layer of struggle if you are trans. The very act of accessing a clinic can be undermining, never mind the pain. 'I spend most days with a hot water bottle and take it everywhere, plus painkillers and cramp pads that I stick on myself, and it makes the dysphoria even worse,' said Dee.

I met Dee while we were filming *The Pill Revolution* with Davina McCall and they are a positive force for good, aiming to replace gender dysphoria with gender euphoria. They have shortish hair (colours vary), big glasses and an ever-changing wardrobe; sometimes they bind their chest, sometimes they don't. Sometimes their hair is up in pretty patterned clasps; sometimes they are on a Pride march in a baggy T-shirt and a baseball cap. Much of this is charted with honesty – and playfulness – on Instagram. When we last spoke, Dee said they were feeling transmasc, on the masculine side of non-binary, but another Instagram post said: 'Today I woke up feeling femme and that scared me,' and they decided to wear hoop earrings and eyeliner. But in the end, Dee concluded: 'Your expression may fluctuate, but you are still trans.' They said they started 'stumbling along different identities and labels – gender-fluid, genderqueer, gender-nonconforming were just a few I looked into . . . but I realised something, you don't NEED a label. You don't need to define yourself or your identity if you don't want to . . . I'm not dropping all labels because non-binary still feels like home to me.' Such fluidity makes forays into contraception somewhat complicated: at the time of writing, Dee had a bisexual partner and used condoms. Dee also, so far, has chosen not to take testosterone.

BEING NON-BINARY ON THE PILL

'I'd been on the pill since I was fourteen or fifteen at school. I was open with my mum and told her. I was in a great committed relationship and having sex. I took Levest [a combined estrogen and progestin pill] for years. Three weeks on, one week's break. At first it was amazing,' said Dee. 'But in my early twenties I started getting headaches every day and I'd wake up in bed feeling nauseous, so I came off it. I really did love routine periods, and I didn't trust barrier methods back then. I had mental health signs that were possibly down to the pill, and I wanted to see who I was without hormones. Coming off the pill, I did have some mental health issues, but not as drastic as being on birth control. Birth control was a darker place mentally.' But the downside was the cramping and chronic pain they now suffer without the combined pill. Healthcare professionals told them to go on contraception again, and they tried the progestin-only pill: 'Me and this pill DID NOT get on and I wanted to share some reasons why I've decided this short romance is OVER,' wrote Dee. 'My chest felt really tender, now this is a totally normal symptom; however, as a Transmasc individual this made me highly uncomfortable. I didn't have these pains prior to taking the mini pill and I didn't like the dysphoria that came with it.' For the moment, Dee remains stuck in a no-man's-land, or perhaps a no-trans-land, in pain with a serious need for more medical investigation – and long waiting lists.

But their battles have brought some wisdom they want to pass on to other trans patients: 'Be vocal about what you need. In terms of gender, you're the expert. Be honest about what you need on the phone beforehand with the surgery and say, "I am a trans individual." Maybe choose a younger doctor too. Tell them you're non-binary and that you use they/them pronouns or whatever you choose.' Dee has been consulting with their local sexual health clinic in Luton, 'making sure it doesn't look gendered.' Trans and non-binary people made up 0.5 per cent of the 2021 UK Census. That's 1 in 200 people, but, said Dee, 'there's such a moral panic around the trans issue we're not going to be a priority any time soon. I just wish doctors would use more neutral rather than gendered language.'

WHAT ARE RELIABLE TRANS SEXUAL HEALTH SOURCES?

There are lots of barriers for trans, non-binary and gender-diverse people accessing contraception and sexual health services, but we will try to overcome at least some of them in this chapter. The hormonal pill does much so more than simply providing contraception – although that's a bonus – and it's a tool trans and non-binary people can use in multiple ways, alongside gender-affirming hormones or just by itself. I've been trawling for evidence-based information on transgender contraception, and while the Wild West of TikTok, Reddit and Instagram is entertaining, occasionally nutty and sometimes worth consulting, one of the more solid medical sources in the UK is the Faculty of Sexual and Reproductive Healthcare's online section 'Contraceptive Choices and Sexual Health for Transgender and Non-Binary People'[1]. It's worth downloading and indeed talking to your doctor for reference. Dr Julia Bailey (she/they) at University College London has written a newer 2023 guidance paper 'Sexual Health Needs of Trans and Non-Binary People',[2] for clinicians, outlining how to 'respond to the needs of trans and non-binary people in ways which are appropriate, affirming and supportive'. This guide covers gender identity, pronouns, transition and contraceptive methods, as well as ways that health services can make people feel welcome, 'and how to ask sexual health questions sensitively without making assumptions about gender, sexuality, anatomy or sexual practice.' The University of

California at San Francisco has really detailed guidelines and research into transcare on its website.[3] But long-term research on the crossover effects of gender-affirming hormones and the synthetic hormones in contraception is lacking, so far.[4]

Very little data and evidence has been gathered – thanks to bias, stigma and the newness of this subject – so there's still a certain amount of learning by trial and error for trans and non-binary contraceptive users and their doctors. There are huge struggles for trans men (assigned female at birth) and trans women (assigned male at birth) in accessing care. Many doctors will never have seen a trans-identifying patient but as Phil Rolland, a consultant gynaecological oncologist who worked on the new trans and gender-diverse care guidance for Royal College of Obstetricians and Gynaecologists, pointed out: 'It's highly likely that if an obstetrician or gynaecologist hasn't already consulted or treated a trans or gender-diverse patient then it is only a matter of time before they do.'[5] The guidance discusses ways to take a non-judgemental sexual and reproductive history from a trans or non-binary patient, the importance of respecting a patients' preferences when it comes to pronouns, titles, names and family relationships, and considering the background of individual well-being and health outcomes. 'Sadly, trans and gender-diverse individuals say they often feel judged and misunderstood by the health service,' said Mr Rolland. 'This can act as a barrier for them when it comes to accessing vital care, and we as healthcare professionals have a role to play in making them feel listened to and recognised.'

For trans and gender-diverse patients, it is worth seeking out the expertise and acceptance of a trans-specific NHS or non-profit clinic in the UK, or the trans-friendly charities like Planned Parenthood across the US. In London, there is the 56T clinic at 56 Dean Street and CliniQ in Denmark Hill; elsewhere there is the Butterfly Clinic at Royal Liverpool Hospital and Clinic T in Brighton. Soho's 56 Dean Street hosts the famous NHS sexual health clinic, which originally opened to serve gay and bisexual men – and it now serves the whole LGBTQI+ community.

There, I found an expert who has consulted with thousands of patients: Dr Tara Suchak, a hardworking pioneer in gender-diverse contraception, a consultant in HIV, and a sexual health and gender specialist. Dr Suchak and I had coffee together for two hours in the staid members' rooms of the British Library, where I was working. Her denim mini-skirt and exquisitely painted nails, plus our graphic conversation, had crusty academics tuning in and twitching into their tweeds. We laughed. 'I'm mixed race, from a working-class background from Newcastle – and everyone thinks I'm a hairdresser,' said Dr Suchak. In fact, her expertise is unparalleled in the UK and her work at 56T is more than full time: 'People are flocking to see us for hormone monitoring, swabs, PReP [the anti-HIV drug] as well as contraception. There are real horror stories in trans healthcare; people have come down to us from Scotland, Yorkshire and Wales, and waited years for help.' Three years ago, Dr Suchak led the team that opened a pilot gender care clinic at Dean Street for patients aged seventeen and over, and she said it is some of the most fulfilling – but tough – work she has ever done. The clinic provides assessment and diagnosis of gender dysphoria, hormone therapy, voice therapy and possible referral for surgery. But quite often, she finds 'people come sometimes with their families, and they've been putting life on hold, not wanting to go into employment or higher education because they don't want to transition during their time there. "I want to go out there as the person I feel inside," they say. They're often struggling with mental health, on all sorts of antidepressants, and instead we give them hormones, which are, as you know, the cheapest of drugs, and they go on to university or whatever. For most, there have been gender dysphoria red flags since childhood and through puberty, and about 80 per cent are already taking hormones, and more do that after seeing us. They come back a year later, and they're often off all the antidepressants and their mental health has improved. It's the story of a wonderful thing, and it does lift you up.' The hormones offered are better-tolerated body-identical injections or rub-in gels. Masculinising testosterone gel for trans men costs the NHS around £1 a day. Feminising hormones for trans women include body-identical estrogen tablets or patches or gels, which are often even cheaper.

WHAT DOES GENDER-AFFIRMING SURGERY INVOLVE?

Although gender-affirming surgery is discussed a lot, economics, access and choice mean only a minority of trans men and women actually have genitourinary surgery – between 4 and 13 per cent, according to limited academic studies,[6] which were mostly American. Chest reduction surgery or breast augmentation is more prevalent, at between 8 and 25 per cent. (Again, samples are small, and the data is difficult to obtain; much is done in the private sector, and surveys are often anonymous and unverifiable.) The majority of people identify as a trans man or woman without surgery, and sometimes even without hormones. So, for many trans and non-binary people still having penis-in-vagina sex, contraception is relevant.

For trans men, as Dr Suchak said: 'Being on testosterone will not necessarily stop you getting pregnant, particularly at first.' For the minority of people who want gender-affirming surgery, it is a serious and expensive operation with life-changing consequences that can affect fertility and sometimes the ability to orgasm, with high complication rates. But the basics are this: trans men who were assigned female at birth and have had a vaginectomy and a hysterectomy to remove the womb (and possibly an oophorectomy to remove the ovaries) will no longer need contraception. The same applies to trans women who have had penile inversion vaginoplasty. In this complex operation, the penis and testicles are removed, and the sensitive skin of the penis is used to create a vaginal cavity. Then the glans is used to simulate a clitoris, while the urethra is shortened. A small minority of trans men also have a phalloplasty: grafted skin usually from the thigh or arm, which is used to create a 'neopenis', which cannot become erect on its own. Others opt for metoidioplasty, an operation to construct a small penis from the clitoris after heavy testosterone therapy, which can slightly enlarge the clitoris.

The Dean Street clinic works with Chelsea and Westminster Hospital on gender-affirming surgery referrals, but there are very few surgeons trained to perform these operations in the UK and the waiting lists are years long. After any gender-affirming operation, everyone may still need to consider contraceptive barrier methods like an internal (vaginal) or external condom (penis) to prevent sexually transmitted diseases.

There's a ton of medical complexity here; every patient is different and making assumptions about surgery and hormones is inappropriate. Fortunately, clinics like Dr Suchak's are safe and sympathetic spaces. In a report in *PinkNews*,[7] when 25-year-old Harry (not his real name) went to 56T for the first time, he found himself amazed that practitioners actually knew how to help him. 'My questions were mainly around whether or not the pill (which I thought must have some kind of hormone in it) would interact with my testosterone, what contraceptives would be available to me other than condoms, and what would be my risks of HIV exposure as a gay trans man.' Harry had asked similar questions at other sexual health clinics, but he was told that he would have to go to a specialist. But at 56T he said: 'They really knew their stuff and made me feel at ease. I was told – through their trans-inclusive practice and approach – that my body wasn't odd, unusual or strange. For the first time, professionals had answers to my questions. That felt really important.' He added: 'In these spaces, you're able to say, as a man with muscles and a beard, "I've had some discoloured, unusual discharge from my vagina" and nobody bats an eyelid. We're treated with the care and attention we deserve.'

Harry's experience is unusual; research in the *British Medical Journal*[8] showed that 'trans people were less likely to have attended a sexual health clinic in the past twelve months compared to cisgender people' and those who did were 'more likely to report experiencing discrimination in a medical setting', as well as high levels of psychological distress. While cis women are less than keen to turn up for cervical smear tests, trans men and non-binary people are even more reluctant, and they need to feel more welcome, understood and included in informational material. Many trans and non-binary people may not even know that smear tests are available to them, although 56T has a no-barriers cervical screening project.[9]

CONTRACEPTION FOR TRANS MEN

I told Dr Suchak that I felt a bit out of my depth in terms of my knowledge of the spectrum of growing gender identifications, but she said: 'Don't worry, I'm always learning. I can't always know all the terms people use. Trans men and trans women, that's fairly clear, but I'm learning that non-binary is not always bang in the middle, and sometimes people experience gender fluidity. It's all about people's lived experience.' And where people go, contraception must follow. For trans men, as Dr Suchak explains, testosterone is not inevitably the solution. 'Some don't like the effects like more body hair and clitoral growth – say if they've previously been sexually abused or had some trauma. They might prefer to build muscle by going to the gym or having protein shakes.'

But what many trans men and non-binary people want to see the back of (like so many of us) is periods, and the progestin-only pill is useful for stopping bleeding, particularly in a higher dose, and can be dropped at any time if there are side effects. Obviously, the combined pill contains estrogen and most trans men don't want that. 'I discuss all the options, and a GP wouldn't have time to go into that kind of detail. I'll even discuss if they want gamete storage [storage of eggs or sperm which is available on the NHS] before starting hormones,' said Dr Suchak. The long-term implant and the Depo-Provera injection are less attractive choices: 'sometimes they get irregular bleeding patterns'. Scrolling around Reddit, I found this contraception story: 'I'm a trans guy and I've had the Nexplanon implant since November and I've basically been bleeding since January. There have been days and weeks in between where I wasn't bleeding, only spotting, but I bleed more days than not. I'm on testosterone and am afraid of an estrogen birth control method possibly messing with my levels. I'm gonna get my T levels tested so going on a different dose of T might make this subside, but I'm just tired and want to keep my options open.'

Testosterone supplementation generally stops periods between two to six months,[10] but fertility can linger on. Patients receiving gonadotrophin-releasing hormone (GnRH) agonists, which suppress ovarian function, should also know there could still be a risk of pregnancy. Some trans men don't want to take a contraceptive pill every day, so Dr Suchak also offers to fit the hormonal coil, which has the advantage of being invisible and forgotten.

Like cervical smears, isn't the coil-fitting frightening and triggering for some? I asked. 'It's a good long-term solution.' After that there's no need to change contraception for up to five years. Dr Suchak added, 'The IUS (coil) is brilliant because sometimes testosterone can convert into estrogen in the body, and the coil provides endometrial protection. Testosterone can also cause vaginal atrophy, so fitting a coil might be painful, and we can offer vaginal estrogen cream for a while beforehand if there's a problem.' Despite cultural assumptions, science shows that hormones are not binary – men and women both naturally have testosterone and estrogen receptors in their bodies. Men make ten times the amount of testosterone women make, but testosterone is still a major female hormone – women in their late teens and early twenties make a larger quantity of testosterone than estrogen, and that slowly declines as they head towards menopause and beyond (the exception is when they are pregnant and estrogen levels are at their highest).[11] We are all more hormonally fluid than we were taught in school.

TRANS MEN, PREGNANCY AND ABORTION

According to a couple of studies, between 40 and 50 per cent of transgender people express desire for future children.[12] When I was an activist a few years ago with Reclaim the Frame, a charity that promoted indie films made by women and people who identify as female, we did cinema screenings with Q&As for *Seahorse*, a moving British documentary directed by Jeanie Finlay about Freddy McConnell, a trans man who gets pregnant. The film opened my eyes to the joys and complexities of this world, but I also wondered about the added trauma for trans men around abortion.

In the US, Planned Parenthood has a regular feed of women talking honestly about their abortion experiences and normalising them on its X and YouTube accounts. 'Hi, my name is Lucky, and I've had an abortion,' said one. I'll bet this story came as a bit of a surprise to the average Twitter user, as it looked as if there was a cis guy on the YouTube video with short hair, glasses and a neat blue jacket with a checked waistcoat. But it turned out Lucky was a trans man, and he explained his choice: 'I get gender-affirming care from Planned Parenthood. I wound up in a very, very difficult relationship and within three months I found out I was pregnant and I was like "Oh no!" My abortion was one of the greatest acts of compassion I have ever committed; it was an easy decision . . . As for the friends I'd told I was trans, they were like, "Get it." Like, "Great, that's your decision." You want to finally begin your life. It was just one of the best decisions I had ever made in my life. I wish more people understood that abortion was healthcare, plain and simple. It's important to talk about abortion in a healthcare setting because I think that when we don't, we see abortion as this very, very uncommon, isolated thing when it's not. It needs to be shared, it needs to be out here . . . I tell my abortion story because I want people to understand it's not just a women's rights issue – it's a people's rights issue.'[13]

THE PILL AND TRANS WOMEN

Because getting trans care can be taboo, or just plain difficult to access, some trans women and non-binary people who lean towards the feminine spectrum start taking the combined estrogen (ethinylestradiol) and progestin contraceptive pill. 'Often they self-medicate and get female friends to get the prescription, a pill like Dianette, and then use it themselves,' said Dr Suchak. Sometimes people take double the dose to increase the estrogenic effect. But there's a risk here. 'We don't recommend the combined pill as first line in trans women over the age of thirty because of the cardiovascular risk of strokes and clots.' She prefers to give patients safer body-identical estrogen gel or patches. The newer contraception pills like Qlaira, Zoely and Drovelis/Nextstellis with body-identical estrogen would also be safer. There's still controversy over giving trans women body-identical progesterone too, which is not presently prescribed at gender clinics, but it can help mood and sleep.

SEX, DRUGS AND CLINIC GOALS

The trans community needs specialist healthcare everywhere, but the Dean Street clinic has added strains. It's always been a safe space for members of the LGBTQI+ community and sex workers to go for sexual healthcare, and it's even busier now. 'There can be complicated crossovers with these needs. We're here to help everyone,' said Dr Suchak. She was worried about the growing rates reported of sexually transmitted diseases in the UK – up 24 per cent[14] and there is a similar growth in the US, with syphilis and gonorrhoea rates both up. The reasons are not clear, but uptake of the HIV-preventative drug PReP has meant that condom use has fallen. Safe sex is not ubiquitous by any means.

Another interview in *PinkNews*[15] detailed the struggles of a trans sex worker with the pseudonym Mandy, who used to commute two hours from Bristol to London to access non-judgemental sexual healthcare. 'When I went to Bristol's central clinic for a sexual health check-up, they told me they "don't know how to deal with people like me,"' she said. 'I even experienced having a student nurse brought in to look at my post-operative vagina.' She wanted to get tested, 'finding clinicians that are able to handle my trans body and my sex work was an uphill struggle', and she pointed out that the two communities are often intrinsically linked. Eventually she found CliniQ, a trans-led sexual health and well-being service in London. 'For us, our genitals are sometimes a source of trauma or difficulty,' continued Mandy, 'and our bodies after surgical intervention don't always operate the same as, or look the same as, their cis counterparts.'

BRAVE, NEW TRANS WORLD

It's a learning experience, not just for investigative outsiders like myself, but for trans insiders too. Social media, when it's good and responsible, can play a huge part in education and explanation – this is not exactly textbook stuff. Yet. Dee, who we heard from at the start of this chapter, wants to bring more joy and confidence to trans and non-binary sex. One of their Instagram posts starts: 'Sex isn't just penis in vagina. For many LGBTQ+ folks, P in V is never on the table. Sometimes a penis isn't involved or penetration isn't something someone wants to engage in.' People may want to avoid vaginal sex and prefer anal sex. Or vice versa. And people with dysphoria may find genital touching upsetting, but Dee points out there are other erogenous zones from ears down to toes. 'The brain is the biggest sexual organ we have . . . Turning on someone's brain is just as important as turning on the rest of their body.'

And there you have it, in the words of pioneers in the gender zone. While healthcare should lead to happiness, and contraception to pleasurable sex, a lot of the patients coming into Dr Suchak's clinic are war-torn. 'They're angry and depressed about being judged, abused in the media, and struggling to find their own path.' The professionals looking after them are equally exhausted. Because mainstream medicine is not yet fully embracing trans care, and the knowledge is limited, a huge burden falls on clinics like Dean Street and their workers. 'I wouldn't make it through without my team, my nurses. They're amazing,' said Dr Suchak. 'Sometimes I just want to retire. I'm really tired and I'm only in my early forties. Trans health care means sleepless nights. But I'm keeping going.' She pauses and smiles. 'I still haven't had time to put up my roller blinds at home.'

CHAPTER ELEVEN

WHY DON'T WE TALK
HONESTLY ABOUT ABORTIONS?

Why don't we talk about abortion together more? Why is abortion such an achingly lonely experience for so many women, when a third of us have one or more in our lifetime?

We need to bring abortion out of the backstreets into the light. Abortion is a necessary and undeniable part of women's healthcare, something that most of us don't plan on, but many of us have to embrace, yet it is steeped in shame and weaponised by politicians.

Despite the sound and fury over abortion bans in America, access to the abortion pill is completely changing the archaic medical landscape, and over half of abortions are self-administered at home.[1] In the UK, the pill is used in more than 80 per cent of terminations, and abortions are the highest they have ever been since legalisation. There are many heartbreaking reasons for abortions, including imperilled maternal or foetal heath, or incest or rape. Those criminal offences often go unpunished, except for the punishment of the pregnant. But it is also clear that there is a seismic shift happening; despite many contraceptive choices, women are not choosing contraception. Abortion is on the rise.

ALMOST HALF OF PREGNANCIES ARE UNINTENDED

The termination rate is at its highest ever in Britain since the Abortion Act of 1967, a rate of 19 per 1,000 women[2] annually, going up to 27 in the most deprived areas of England, and 16 per 1,000 in Scotland.[3] Meanwhile in the US, abortions were estimated at 14 per 1,000,[4] and despite new draconian restrictions in some states after the overturning of Roe v. Wade in 2022, abortions are still on the rise as women cross state lines or buy pills by post.[5] Perhaps the convenience of the pill increases the willingness of women and their partners to go ahead with abortions, and reduces worry about the risks of unintended conception. But there is another trend: abortion providers are citing the growing numbers of slightly older women coming in who realise they just can't make ends meet for their family if they have another child. Plus, there's a new questioning of hormonal contraception, a lack of access to other contraceptive choices, and a move to less effective rhythm methods.

Over the last decade, around 45 per cent of pregnancies in the US and UK have been unintended.[6] One-third of women have had an abortion during their lifetime in the UK,[7] a quarter in America.[8] A recent survey showed 90 per cent of adults in the UK were pro-choice.[9] Many of us, including me, have had more than one abortion over almost forty years of reproductive life. As I and almost everyone I know can attest, contraception is rarely perfect.

PREGNANT AT PRIMARY SCHOOL

As periods and puberty come earlier and earlier,[10] particularly in the US, where some girls are developing breast buds at seven or eight and getting their periods at elementary school, the need to provide safeguarding, early contraceptive education and safe access to abortion is an even bigger responsibility. The head-in-the-sand attitude won't cut it. When I worked as a reporter for *The Times* in the US, long before I was a mother myself, I was sent to report on a young mothers' centre, part of a school in San Jose, where girls who had got pregnant as young as eleven or twelve were able to keep their babies in a nursery next door to the classroom where they attended their lessons. I spent time with the girls — funny, confident, sensible, many of them thirteen or fourteen years old with their own toddlers by then — and I wanted to cry: they were babies having babies. Now that I've had children myself, I realise how much weightier and long-lasting their burdens were, and perhaps they didn't yet have a full sense of that. You'll do anything for this small person: stay up all night for it, fight for it, curb your career for it, lay down your life for it. It's a beautiful abnegation of self. And these girls were doing this often before they were teenagers themselves. Most of them came from economically deprived backgrounds and were Black or Latina, the very groups that have the worst access to contraception and abortion in the American healthcare system.

In an essay in the *New York Times*, writer and editor Nicole Walker wrote about her abortion, aged eleven, after she was 'impregnated by my fourteen-year-old babysitter'.[11] If she hadn't had the abortion, she writes, 'My life would not have been my own. I would be a prisoner subject to a body's whims – and not *my* body's whims, but the whims of a teenage boy, who, as best I can tell, experienced no consequences for inflicting what his body wanted upon my own.'

At that time, abortion was legal where she lived in Utah, but Nicole said: 'I did not feel lucky to get an abortion. I felt like garbage. The babysitter did not have to go to the clinic. The babysitter was not shunned and censured by our community. Most people didn't even know what he had done, though they seemed to know something bad had happened to me – or perhaps that I had done something wrong. Only my mom and I were subject to the shame of entering that special building for that special procedure.'

A CONDOM CRUMPLED, A DIAPHRAGM DISPLACED . . .

That 'special procedure', a surgical abortion, must have been beyond terrifying at Nicole's age; anyone of any age still finds it tough. I've had two surgical abortions – one in my mid-twenties, when I was single, and another in my early thirties, months after I had my first baby, and couldn't cope with another one so quickly. Both my abortions were the result of failed contraception — a condom crumpled, a diaphragm displaced. I am lucky enough now to have three fantastic grown-up children, and I frame my abortions as late contraception, caused by a combination of human error, chance and birth control methods which were decidedly old-fashioned. That mirrors the feelings of the majority of women about abortion. A study of almost seven hundred women across America showed that 95 per cent felt afterwards that termination was the right decision, and experienced decreasing emotional intensity over time.[12]

Because I didn't want to use hormonal contraception, I increased my chances of unintentional conception. Diaphragms have a failure rate of 12 per cent a year with typical use, and condoms have a failure rate of 15 per cent.[13] Actually, when I think about it, I had a huge success rate with the diaphragm and spermicidal gel combined over ten years, with just that one slip-up. By the time I was twenty-five, I'd seen two of my girlfriends through surgical abortions, so I knew what to do when my own turn came. I knew about taking to bed, tears of relief and agony, supplies of sanitary pads, paracetamol and hot water bottles, but I remember what actually worked best afterwards for one of my friends at university was talking into the night and smoking a couple of joints to get through the cramps.

CAN WE HELP MAKE ABORTION A WOMAN'S CHOICE — AND A SHARED CONVERSATION?

I found myself pregnant after a drunk one-night stand where no one stayed the night. After some fumbling I realised the condom was in me, and not on him. 'I'm sure it will be fine,' I said, and we remained friends. I had such hard, painful tits within a few weeks I knew it was barely worth splashing out on a pregnancy test, but the grim blue line duly appeared, and I called the local clinic for an appointment. I never told the man I'd had sex with that I was pregnant. What's the point of him going through that when we're not together, I thought then. I didn't really want sympathy, or a debate, or any palaver. I had a full-time job to do, and I just wanted this over with as quickly and quietly as possible.

I rang an experienced girlfriend. She said: 'Of course, I'll pick you up afterwards in a taxi.' I firmly believe in a woman's right to choose abortion, and to choose who she tells about her abortion. Our bodies, ourselves. Obviously, some women dare not tell of their abortion for their own safety in an abusive or secret relationship, and some just don't want the complicated conversation, but I also wonder writing this now how many millions of kind, empathetic men out there have no idea their sexual partner has had an abortion. Maybe secrecy like mine is doing us no favours in starting to normalise abortion for men too.

There were only surgical abortions then, before the abortion pill was licensed in the UK in 1991, so I went to one of the big independent London clinics and got an appointment. I remember very little about the operation (it was vacuum aspiration) other than waking up in a ward and then walking out to the taxi with a giant, cardboardy sanitary pad between my legs. I only took one day off work; it was an early termination, around eight weeks, and the cramps were bearable. I felt incredibly relieved, like I'd crawled out from under a heavy stone. I had an easy experience, thanks to the British Pregnancy Advisory Service. They and MSI Reproductive Choices provide many of the abortions for the National Health Service in the UK now. But what's it like looking after women like me? What actually happens during a surgical abortion?

SURGICAL ABORTION

Dr Yvonne Neubauer is the UK Associate Clinical Director for Surgical Abortion at MSI Reproductive Choices, and I talked to her after a long day on the front line in their Bristol Treatment Centre. Like all the MSI clinics, it has signature turquoise blue doors and the symbol of the charity is an open door. (Now that legal buffer zones have been agreed to prevent protests within 150 metres of clinics, doctors and vulnerable patients will no longer have to run the gauntlet of occasional demonstrations by anti-abortion protest groups to reach the safety of that door.) On an average day, Dr Neubauer will probably operate on sixteen or seventeen women who need surgical abortions, mostly free and funded by the NHS. She started off her training in obstetrics and gynaecology with the NHS before she moved to MSI Reproductive Choices. 'We didn't get any abortion training,' she said of her official medical education. 'We covered the surgical management of miscarriage but abortion care was not part of our early curriculum.'

Dr Jayne Kavanagh of University College London is the Clinical Education Lead for the Royal College of Obstetrics and Gynaecology's Making Abortion Safe programme, and said: 'When abortion is taught, it is often focused on ethical and legal aspects, rather than on clinical training, further stigmatising it as an unusual or controversial subject rather than essential healthcare. The same is true for postgraduate training, even for fields such as obstetrics and gynaecology.'[4] Dr Neubauer learned on the job, but it is disturbing how often training in women's health, like abortion and menopause, is left up to chance in work placements, and she now campaigns for abortion training to be part of the compulsory core curriculum for obstetrics and gynaecology students. Presently the basics are taught, but the Advanced Skills Module in Abortion Care is optional.

At the MSI clinic, the initial counselling and preparing is done by nurses and midwives, so Dr Neubauer usually meets the women for the first time on the day of their procedure. There's a real warmth about her, and dedication. 'I'm in clinic at 8am, ready to go. There are women looking at you in your uniform scrubs, and for some it might be a tearful, emotional time so you take them aside and chat about what they're worried about, their doubts. Sometimes they decide it's not for them today. I say, "Let us know and come back if you want." It can be a really overwhelming feeling for them, and we respect that.'

How does surgical abortion work?

At MSI, medical abortion with pills is available up to nine weeks and six days, and over ten weeks abortions are surgical, but it also depends on medical history and people can choose to have a surgical abortion earlier anyway. The cut-off point in British law for all abortions is twenty-three weeks and six days. Abortions may be performed after twenty-four weeks in certain circumstances, for example, if the mother's life is at risk or the child would be born severely disabled. Dr Neubauer handles surgical abortions for low-risk patients. 'If there's risk of comorbidity [another health condition], I arrange a referral to an NHS hospital.' Women who are further along usually come in overnight for clinical preparation and doctors use dilators to prepare and soften the cervix.

Later abortions up to twenty weeks sometimes weigh very differently on women, but they are only 1 per cent of the total, and only 0.1 per cent of abortions are after twenty-four weeks.[15] The quickest procedures are six or seven-week vacuum aspirations that gently suction out the pregnancy and take around five minutes. A local anaesthetic or continuous sedation, where the patient is conscious but relaxed and relatively pain-free, can be used. More complicated operations involve dilation and evacuation that could require forceps, and might last fifteen to twenty minutes, with the patient under a general anaesthetic. 'The doctor makes every effort to ensure the procedure is complete and the uterus is empty,' said Dr Neubauer. 'We also advise patients to complete a short course of antibiotics afterwards to reduce the risk of infection.'

Depending on each patient, bleeding can last for one to two weeks and will be similar to a heavy period, although any larger blood clots warrant going back to the doctor. Cramping pains are also normal following the procedure, as the womb returns to its normal size, and the doctors advise on appropriate pain relief to take. Sometimes women are shocked by the amount of pain and bleeding. 'The better the patient is informed, the easier it is to deal with,' said Dr Neubauer.

She finds the long day operating is both physically and emotionally draining. 'But I feel like I'm making a difference.' Whatever the timescale and difficulty, Dr Neubauer (and indeed, everyone I met at MSI Reproductive Choices) is completely non-judgemental. 'Abortion is an essential part of healthcare, and there should be no stigma around it. People give such a range of reasons, from not being able to see their GP to get the contraception they want, and some just don't get on with the side effects. They'll also say, 'I just can't afford to be pregnant' or 'I just can't afford to expand my family'. We're seeing more older women coming in now, although teenage pregnancy is down. It comes back round to access to contraception.'

ENTER THE ABORTION PILL

Thank heaven for the abortion pill, which in the US is at least eliminating the need for humiliating marches into abortion clinics, particularly when there are protestors harassing the patients outside. In the UK, almost all abortions up until ten weeks are done by taking two pills: mifepristone, which stops the supply of hormones to the womb, and then misoprostol, which induces the abortion. It has a great safety record – an analysis of over a hundred scientific studies over thirty years, shows that 99 per cent of women had a complication-free experience, and in the UK to be extra safe, women who might have other possible risks or conditions are asked to come in for a scan first.

It's worth mentioning here that one in ninety of all pregnancies are ectopic,[16] and that can affect the outcome. My friend Rebecca Cheshire, who is a senior nurse in emergency Obstetrics and Gynaecology at the Royal Free Hospital in London, sees occasional cases of ectopic pregnancies continuing after the double abortion pill is used. 'Women come in in severe pain or still bleeding three weeks later, and when we scan them we see the ectopic pregnancy in their tubes.' If there's little pain, they monitor to see if the pregnancy will discharge itself due to lack of hormones, but often they have to operate, which can cause scarring or the loss of one of the two fallopian tubes. MSI uses clinical history and ultrasound to assess the risk of ectopic pregnancy and advise patients on whether they need to seek medical help to rule out an ectopic pregnancy.

How easy is it to get the abortion pill in the UK?

Maya Oppenheim is the women's correspondent at the *Independent*, an online newspaper in the UK with a large circulation, as well as the author of *The Pocket Guide to the Patriarchy*. Maya decided to go public about her experience with the abortion pill in 2022[17] with a devastatingly honest article. She also talked to me more recently in London about the extraordinary reaction her tell-it-like-it-is account received on social media from women. 'There were a few trolls, but just so many messages of support. Women just found the honesty really helpful.'

When Maya discovered she was pregnant – peeing on the test stick in the less-than-ideal location of the toilets at Westfield Shopping Centre – she knew she could not keep the baby. 'Despite being in a relationship, I didn't feel mentally, financially or logistically ready,' she said. At the moment, work and career mattered to Maya more than starting a family; over half of women in the UK do not get pregnant under the age of thirty. Mothers are getting older, the economics are getting tighter, and freedom is prized for longer. She decided to have a medical abortion using the two pills.

However, getting an appointment to have the pills prescribed turned out to be more complicated than Maya expected. A call to her local NHS hospital went unanswered, so she tried the British Pregnancy Advisory Service charity. They were 'currently experiencing exceptionally high call volumes', so she waited for a long time, 'with the soothing music playing on the end of the line having the opposite effect to what they intended.' In the end, Maya gave up and sent an email instead. The wait was nerve-wracking. Two days later, the BPAS called and said she would have to wait three weeks for a phone consultation. 'That meant I wouldn't be able to have the actual abortion until a month after requesting it. That would've left me just a couple of weeks away from the ten-week cut-off point for a medical abortion, which involves taking two pills. I didn't want to have a surgical abortion after ten weeks.'

The NHS website says you should not have to wait more than two weeks from when you first contact an abortion provider to having an abortion, but theory is different from practice. 'The man on the phone admitted the BPAS was grappling with massive delays, receiving 1,000 requests for abortions a day. I stated the obvious – that this was a time-sensitive procedure, and I wasn't willing to wait that long – and he said I could have a phone consultation for an abortion a week later. But if I wanted something sooner, I was told I'd have to travel hundreds of miles to Doncaster or Liverpool for an in-person appointment. This was beginning to feel like a nightmare.'

Maya then called another women's health charity, MSI Reproductive Choices UK, which managed to give her a telephone consultation that evening. 'I explained I'd had a minuscule amount of discharge, which triggered a request to come in for an in-person appointment and a scan, rather than simply sending the abortion pills in the post.' Pills became available by post with a telephone consultation during the Covid pandemic. Previously, women had to take the first pill, mifepristone, at a clinic. 'I was offered a consultation in Central London a week later, but I ended up opting for an appointment in the small Kent village of Aylesham, a five-hour trip, but it meant I would be seen a few days earlier. My granny had died a couple of days before I'd found out I was pregnant, and I couldn't face the prospect of being in too much pain to attend her funeral.' At the Kent clinic, the ultrasound showed Maya was six and a half weeks pregnant – further along than she had thought.

What's it like taking the abortion pill?

Maya took the first abortion pill, mifepristone, on the train back to London. 'I was relieved there were no side effects. If you throw up within an hour, you have to let the doctors know, as the pill may not be effective. That evening I did feel a little strange, but it was when I took the second abortion pill twenty-four hours later that the all-consuming agony hit: the worst pain I remember feeling in my life.'

The medical staff had been supportive, but no one had explained to Maya quite how painful an early medical abortion could be. 'I chose to put the second pill in my mouth for thirty minutes, rather than the much scarier option of inserting it into my vagina. The pill pretty much wholly dissolved in my mouth in twenty minutes. Before long, I was writhing on the floor in pain, with paracetamol and ibuprofen scattered around me. No matter how I positioned myself or where I placed a cushion, there was no way to get comfortable or escape the cramps. I must have gone to the toilet about thirty times in the space of three hours, partly as a way to distract myself from the deep, roaring pain.'

As she crawled out of the toilet, groaning and in too much pain to even sit up and drink water, Maya kept wondering if what she was experiencing was normal, and she started panicking about the nurse's warning about severe bleeding. 'They said go to the hospital if I soak through two sanitary pads in an hour and blood is "pouring out like urine".' Fortunately, that didn't happen, 'but that didn't stop me from incessantly checking to ensure I was not about to bleed to death'. After three hours, the pain did abruptly subside. 'The feeling was reminiscent of a sea of calm after a violent storm,' said Maya. She also said she was staggered at the difference between the official guidance on the pain, and the hellish reality of it. 'I would rather have been prepared properly for the pain, but it's still so taboo to give us this information.'

She had some bleeding over the next few days, and was told to avoid sex, baths, sports and tampons for a while. 'I'm deeply relieved I'm no longer pregnant, and massively grateful I live in a country where abortions are legal. But this relief is bittersweet due to my disappointment and shock at how poor abortion provision is in the UK, and how much better it could be.' We also need to note here that Maya's experience is not what everyone finds taking the abortion pill – many women have a much less uncomfortable time, and it's a very safe option.

WHY IS ABORTION A POSTCODE-LOTTERY?

At least Maya was in London. In Scotland, if the wait goes beyond the legal limit for a pill termination, there is nowhere to get a surgical abortion and women have to travel to England. Dr Neubauer says women come miles for the procedure at her MSI clinic in Bristol, as there is no access to care in many more rural areas. 'People get up at 5am to get a train from Plymouth or Exeter to get here on time, and then there's a long journey back,' said Dr Neubauer. Abortion is unavailable after ten weeks in Northern Ireland, thirteen weeks in Scotland, and late-term surgical abortions are unavailable in Wales, so all those women have to travel to England for operations.

'Considering it's one of the most common gynaecological operations, it should be available in every part of the UK,' said Elizabeth Walden, director of global communications at MSI Reproductive Choices. At least it's available somehow here; in the US, twenty-four states now have abortion bans.[18] Women travel thousands of miles and cross state lines, at their own expense, for help. Unless they can get abortion pills illegally and secretly posted to them, the women in the states with abortion bans are left behind. 1 in 5 cross state lines for help.

ABORTION IN FRANCE

My second abortion took place in France, where I had been sent alongside my then husband, who was a foreign correspondent for *The Times*, to work as a columnist in the Paris office of the newspaper. We had just had our first baby and were mired equally in delight about him, and grief for my husband's father who had died in an accident the month before the birth. It was a difficult time. My son was rushed back into hospital a few days after he was born, and I struggled to breastfeed him properly. In the end, we resorted to bottles of formula, and he started thriving.

When I realised I might be pregnant in our first month

living in Paris, a first failure for the trusty diaphragm that had worked for years, I couldn't cope. I'd gone to get the morning-after pill, but it was too late, after ovulation in my cycle. Additionally, our adorable eight-month-old son seemed to have no intention of sleeping through the night and he could crawl at speed on his belly like a sniper during the day. On contract with *The Times*, I didn't get staff maternity leave, so I'd only taken a month off work. Back at work part-time, I was exhausted, despite also having a part-time au pair.

I discussed the situation with my sympathetic husband. I pre-armed myself with medical vocabulary which had, inconveniently, not been in my Scottish Higher French at school. I went to my elegant, immaculately coiffed doctor in the 7th Arrondissement, and said: 'Je voudrais un avor-tement.' Madame le docteur nodded and could not have been more helpful. She would call the clinic straightaway. Seeing that I looked a bit stressed, she also recommended a very good local restaurant and wrote its name on her prescription pad. *Vive la France*!

This was a much better abortion experience, partly because the French medical system is so good, and there was no feeling whatsoever that anyone was judging me. I arrived at a clinic in a smart part of Paris, where the male ob-gyn looked like an actor from a hospital soap. He stroked me reassuringly and a tad creepily on the shoulder as I counted down from the anaesthetic: '10-9-8-7-6 . . .' and out. I awoke in a private room with leafy trees tap-ping the window, and again felt an enormous flood of relief. Plus, compared to my recent thirty-two hours in childbirth, the cramps were nothing. Some weeks later, we went to the restaurant the doctor recommended. Looking back, if I'd been courageous, I would have written the abortion story up in my Paris diary, which appeared every week in *The Saturday Times Magazine*. Instead, I told no one.

Of course, of all the places in the world, France was exactly where abortion was no longer a dirty word, despite the country's Catholic roots. French feminists have a long tradition of going public about their abortions. That began in April 1971, when 343 women, including writers like Simone de Beauvoir and Françoise Sagan, actors like Catherine Deneuve, as well as singers and philosophers, all made a statement of 'MeToo' (long before hashtags and social media) about their own abortions. De Beauvoir penned the call to arms to overturn the anti-abortion laws:

'One million women in France have abortions every year. Condemned to secrecy, they do so in dangerous conditions – while under medical supervision, this is one of the simplest procedures. Society is silencing these millions of women. I declare that I am one of them. I declare that I have had an abortion. Just as we demand free access to contraception, we demand the freedom to have an abortion.'[19]

The feminist abortion confession statement was also signed by one of my heroes, the great director Agnès Varda, who made the 1976 film *One Sings, the Other Doesn't* about trying to obtain an abortion in France in 1962. Until 1974, abortion remained a crime, encoded way back by Emperor Napoleon Bonaparte, but the last execution for an abortion-related crime in France was in 1943. When Paris was under the pro-Nazi Vichy regime, 39-year-old

Marie-Louise Giraud was guillotined on the morning of 30 July in the courtyard of the Prison de la Roquette, for having performed twenty-seven abortions on women in the Cherbourg area of France. (Giraud became a feminist hero and Isabelle Huppert later played her in a 1988 film *Story of Women*.)

Three years after the 343 outed themselves, the law was changed and the *faiseuses d'anges* – the 'angel makers', the name given to the women who provided illegal backstreet abortions – were no longer needed. That's still not the case elsewhere today. The World Health Organization estimates that there are 73 million abortions[20] round the world each year and around 45 per cent of these are 'unsafe', causing thousands of deaths from complications.[21] One of the leaders of the French 343, Marie-Jo Bonnet, a feminist historian, told *TIME* magazine: 'Women's bodies are our territory, and it's a territory that has been colonised by the power of men. It is an emancipation. We are taking back the power of our own lives.'[22]

MEANWHILE, IN THE LAND OF THE FREE . . .

The British and French abortion revolutions were over half a century ago, yet here we are back at abortion ground zero again in America, and American feminists are speaking out, just as the French did. In some of the states that have banned abortion, doctors risk life in prison for providing terminations. How can that possibly be? Because American women's bodies were recolonised in 2022 and choice wrenched away from them, after the

Republican-controlled Supreme Court reversed the Roe v. Wade decision of 1973, which had made abortion a constitutional right. At that moment, Margaret Atwood's feminist dystopian classic *The Handmaid's Tale* transmogrified from a book to a television series to actual American law. Now that each individual state could dictate what women did with their bodies, enforced motherhood was a possibility. Thus began a sustained attempt by anti-abortion campaigners to force state legislatures to restrict abortion rights, including criminal penalties for doctors performing terminations. This continues, despite the fact that 62 per cent of Americans in a 2022 survey[23] believed abortion should be legal, and that went up to 66 per cent support among women only. Even 60 per cent of Catholics supported abortion rights; the only refuseniks listed in that survey were 'white evangelicals' and a majority of Republicans.

As Atwood wrote in the *Guardian* after American women lost the constitutional right to abortion, 'Women who cannot make their own decisions about whether or not to have babies are enslaved, because the state claims ownership of their bodies and the right to dictate the use to which their bodies must be put. The only similar circumstance for men is conscription into an army. In both cases there is risk to the individual's life, but an army conscript is at least provided with food, clothing, and lodging.'[24]

The situation is crazy: a country whose majority firmly believes in safe abortion is watching rights being torn away from women, state by state. Most abortions are now banned in twenty-four 'red' Republican states, particularly in the south. Louisiana, Texas, Tennessee, West Virginia, South Dakota, Oklahoma, Kentucky, Arkansas and Alabama have taken a particularly hard line, with no exceptions for rape or incest.[25] At time of writing, seventeen states and the District of Columbia allow abortion, and the rest have restrictions. I remember the Tweet the abortion charity Planned Parenthood put out on the day Roe v. Wade was overturned and looked it up: 'BREAKING: The Supreme Court just overturned Roe v. Wade, ending our constitutional right to abortion. We know you may be feeling a lot of things right now – hurt, anger, confusion. Whatever you feel is OK. We're here with you – and we'll never stop fighting for you.'

Let's be clear: this ban falls disproportionately on the economically deprived who are already struggling for food, clothing and lodging, and cannot afford to take a plane or a train to a nearby liberal state to acquire the abortion pill or a termination, and who cannot afford to raise another child. The ban falls harder on minorities too – a recent survey showed nearly half of Asian Americans said they did not know where to access abortion medication if they needed it.[26] In fact, there is an 'underground railroad' anonymously posting abortion pills out to women in states with bans, and several websites based outside the US that send out mifepristone and misoprostol, the two pills used in a medical abortion. This, despite anti-abortion campaigners in some states trying to use the 1873 Comstock Act – an archaic law designed to prevent the dissemination of pornography, 'lewd' writings and any 'instrument, substance, drug, medicine, or thing' that could be used in an abortion – to prevent pill postage.

The *New York Times* estimated that there had been at least 50,000 pill doses sent to women in the first six months of the abortion ban.[27] Planned Parenthood has worked to encourage abortions by telemedicine and launched a defence fund to support legal challenges to the new anti-abortion laws being pushed through state legislatures. Planned Parenthood warned that some women had been taken in by adverts for 'Crisis Pregnancy Centers', which are anti-choice clinics, where women are dissuaded from having a termination.

In Texas, strict interpretation of the abortion ban has left doctors terrified to help women whose pregnancies are endangering their health and lives. In that state, doctors risk life in prison and fines of up to $100,000 for performing abortions, but that has forced women with obstetrical emergencies into limbo. Babies with serious foetal abnormalities are being carried to full term, despite the gruelling horror for the mother. Samantha Casiano, aged twenty-nine, found out halfway through her pregnancy that her baby had anencephaly and was missing much of her skull and brain. Samantha had to carry her daughter for months. The child died four hours after she was born. 'I was so full of heartbreak and sadness,' she told journalists.[28] A group of women, with circumstances like Samantha, who were unreasonably refused terminations when their or their baby's health was at risk, have taken a lawsuit to ask for clarity in Texas law as to when abortions can be provided under the 'medical emergency' exception, and a judge has made an interim ruling allowing abortions in cases of medical emergencies and fatal foetal diagnoses while litigation continues.

OUR BODIES IN BALLOT BOXES

The story of the loss of abortion rights in the US, and the political and legal battle to regain them, demonstrates how politics can suddenly impact up close on our bodies. We must guard against further inroads by the anti-abortion movement, which is increasingly an anti-contraception movement too, across the world. Look at TikTok, and you will see how cleverly this well-funded campaign is being directed towards the women of Gen Z, with either horror-movie-murder content around abortion, or 'wellness' influencers talking about the dangers of taking pills and the joys of natural fertility cycles as contraception. As we have seen earlier, apps like Natural Cycles say the failure rate with normal use is 7 per cent, and experts at Contraception Choices say around a quarter of women get pregnant using fertility awareness.[29] So, it's more bagatelle than contraception.

The legal situation across various American states changes almost weekly, but this retrograde ban is bringing women and men together in a massive movement across the country. In the 2022 midterm elections, Americans sent a powerful political signal about their unhappiness with abortion law and voted in state ballots to preserve access, even in Republican-dominated areas. Planned Parenthood's 'We Will Not Go Back' campaign mobilised activists at rallies, marches and on social media, and the Center for Reproductive Rights launched legal challenges to the most extreme new anti-abortion laws. What's always worth remembering here for younger activists is that fighting for freedom on TikTok is great, but what really matters is ballot papers and campaigning on the ground, even joining a political party. Only 48 per cent of 18–24-year-olds voted in the last American election (with increasing numbers of Black, Asian and Hispanic voters turning out), but the 52 per cent who are presently disengaged or disenfranchised could make a huge difference to the average woman who gets an abortion in her twenties.

Abortion is also the only part of British healthcare governed under criminal law (after a long struggle it is now decriminalised in Northern Ireland). The British Abortion Act 1967 made it legal to perform abortions within the 24-week limit so long as two doctors sign agreeing that specific criteria are met, but abortion actually remains a criminal offence under the Offences Against the Person Act – from 1861, long before women even had the vote.

In 2023, in the legal case R v. Carla Foster, 44-year-old Carla was imprisoned for using the abortion pill after the time limit of twenty-four weeks, and her child was stillborn at what was estimated between thirty-two and thirty-four weeks. The police examined the Google searches on her phone when she had checked on whether abortions were available after twenty-four weeks, and this provided evidence that she knew how pregnant she was. (Be warned: clearly our health data is not our own;

as mentioned previously, the Flo period-tracking app also shared users' health data with Facebook.[30]) Carla's desperation reflects her complicated circumstances. These tragic events happened in the first few isolated, panicked months of lockdown in 2020, when it was almost impossible to get a doctor's appointment in the pandemic, and the law was changed to make abortion pills available under the ten-week limit by post. It turned out that due to lockdown, Carla had returned to live with her estranged partner and their three sons, but she was secretly pregnant by another man and tried to hide it for as long as she could. Everything seemed to be conspiring against her.

This is what The Hon Mr Justice Pepperall said in his summing up, addressing Carla: 'I accept that you feel very deep and genuine remorse for your actions. You are wracked by guilt and have suffered depression. I accept that you had a very deep emotional attachment to your unborn child and that you are plagued by nightmares and flashbacks seeing your dead child's face. I also take into account the fact you are a good mother to three children who would suffer from your imprisonment. One of your children himself has special needs which means that he is particularly reliant upon your love and support.' And then – almost as though he hadn't heard the humanity in his own words – the judge handed down a 28-month sentence, half of which was to be served in prison. There is no mandatory sentence for abortion, and he could have made the sentence non-custodial. Carla's three children would be left without a mother for over a year. She was taken to jail, but within a month, the Court of Appeal overruled the decision and reduced the term to a fourteen-month suspended sentence. The appeal judge, Dame Victoria Sharp, said: 'It is a case that calls for compassion, not punishment.'

The Faculty of Sexual and Reproductive Healthcare, women's health charities, abortion providers and lawyers are campaigning to get the archaic laws that criminalise abortion removed. The Women's Equality Party (WEP) said: 'The criminalisation of abortion does nothing at all to protect children, all it does is put women at risk. Abortion is healthcare and it must be free, safe and legal . . . Carla's case is a damning indictment of abortion law in England, which criminalises women for simply seeking healthcare. Nothing about this conviction serves the public interest, or the interests of her and her children.'[31]

The WEP also pointed out that in the twenty-first century, women should be able to make their own decisions about abortion – and we don't need a committee, particularly when we are dealing with the simpler abortion pill. Dr Neubauer agrees, throwing up her hands in exasperation. 'Why do we need *two* doctors to say a woman can make her own decision in this area of her life?' There is pressure to scrap the 1967 'two-doctors rule' for authorising abortion in Britain, and a recent article in the *British Medical Journal* said that The Shaping Abortion for Change study, led by the London School of Hygiene and Tropical Medicine, recommended allowing nurses and midwives to authorise an abortion, prescribe abortion drugs, and perform vacuum aspirations as they do in miscarriage care. Isn't it strange that exactly the same procedure is considered 'healthcare' in miscarriage, but a 'crime' in abortion? What century are we in?

THE CELEBRITY PRO-CHOICE ALGORITHM

While getting to the ballot box is the first-line solution, one must not discount — following the rise of a celebrity president like Donald Trump — the power of the celebrity algorithm in this battle over our bodies. When Roe v. Wade was overturned, a chorus of the famous spoke out in support of abortion rights. Actor and writer Lena Dunham tweeted, 'We will not go back. We will fight for our reproductive freedom and stand with those who need us most.' Singer Miley Cyrus posted on Instagram, 'My body, my choice. This is not up for debate.' Comedian Sarah Silverman joked, 'It's just like the Bible says: If you can't control a woman's body, how are you going to control your constituents?' Actress and producer Rashida Jones wrote in an op-ed, 'I don't see how you can be an advocate for women and not be an advocate for reproductive rights.'

Like the French feminists over half a century ago, musicians from Nicki Minaj to Lil' Kim have spoken out freely about their abortion experiences. British singer Lily Allen wrote on Instagram, 'I wish people would stop posting examples of exceptional reasons for having abortions. Most people I know, myself included, just didn't want to have a f***ing baby. And that is reason enough! We don't have to justify it.'[32] Joan Collins, Whoopi Goldberg, Uma Thurman and designer Donna Karan have joined the pro-choice confessional chorus. Comedian Hannah Gadsby wrote, 'I was assaulted, raped and very, very vulnerable. How was I going to raise a child? I would have ended up dead. How is that pro-life?' The experiences of ordinary women are highlighted daily on Twitter accounts like Shout Your Abortion: 'Our stories are ours to tell. This is not a debate.' Planned Parenthood also encourages women, non-binary and trans people to share videos on social media about their abortions. It's necessary, not just to make women feel more comfortable, but to take some of the social media airspace from the well-organised anti-abortion movement.

FROM HELL TO HEALTHCARE

Why don't we swab away the stigma and soothe the pain with our words, our stories and our movies? Honesty must replace shame, or we will never move forward. In all these stories of pain and liberation, what comes through most is the sense of gruelling struggle, a struggle that somehow continues over half a century after abortion was largely legalised across the UK and US. Right now, it feels as though we are backsliding in time, no longer allowed to choose the moment and circumstances when we make the people of the future. We can only hope that in this moment of crisis, at the bottom of the U-bend in abortion care in the US, that we will go in fighting harder than ever before, and that we will go on speaking out. Women like Maya and I are privileged, and our abortion stories are among the least difficult, compared to the suffering and uncertainty many other women go through. But I am glad we shared them. Share yours. Tell your daughters, tell your mothers, tell your friends. Abortion shouldn't be hellish; it should simply be part of healthcare for women.

CHAPTER TWELVE

THE DARK HISTORY OF THE PILL

'I still feel, as I have felt from the first, that there is nothing more important than birth control. I do indeed appreciate the terrific, and unfair struggle,' wrote Katharine Dexter McCormick, the woman who almost single-handedly financed research into the contraceptive pill and the first human trials in the 1950s. You probably won't have heard of her, but you may have heard of Dr John Rock and Dr Gregory Pincus, the male scientists to whom she gave $2m (worth $23m now), as well as $5m to Planned Parenthood to continue the work. Dr Rock and Dr Pincus are credited as the fathers of the pill and led the research, but McCormick's philanthropy made her the mother of invention, in tandem with the controversial birth control pioneer Margaret Sanger. This group of eccentrics presided over experimentation that was scientifically revolutionary – and deeply unethical.

Back in the fifties, the big pharmaceutical companies refused to research and test the early versions of the pill on American women because birth control was far too culturally controversial. Plus, there were legal hurdles, like the Comstock Law of 1873, which lumped contraception in with pornography and prevented its sale and distribution as 'obscene' material. Thus, much of the action around the creation of the pill took place outside of the US.

A team of scientists in Mexico, led by novelist, playwright and scientist Carl Djerassi, synthesised norethindrone progestin from yams in 1951, a step up from previous hormones synthesised from animals that were far too expensive to produce on a mass scale. A similar progestin, norethynodrel, was developed in 1953. The American pharmaceutical company G.D. Searle held the patent for it, and quietly handed supplies of the drug over to Dr Rock and Dr Pincus. But Searle didn't want to get its hands dirty with conducting actual human trials, so the experimental money had to come from private funds, specifically the capacious purse of McCormick.

Usefully, McCormick married into a fortune, but she also came from a well-to-do family and was herself a scientist, the first female graduate in biology from the Massachusetts Institute of Technology in 1904. She became a leading feminist in the early suffrage movement, too. In photographs, she is equally likely to wear a feather boa or a Votes for Women sash. While McCormick the scientist and philanthropist is airbrushed away in earlier histories of the pill, she was both a catalyst and a collaborator, along with Dr Rock, Dr Pincus and Sanger, in bringing it to the world. She was also complicit with them in experiments of a far grimmer nature, which were carried out on the people used as guinea pigs for the first hormonal contraceptives. As we shall hear later, some of the earliest recipients of these progestins were unwitting patients in an American state insane asylum and impoverished Black women in Puerto Rico. The pill pioneers were as unscrupulous as they were unstoppable.

THE WOMEN BEHIND THE MEN BEHIND THE PILL

Reading the pill's history requires employing a sort of Orwellian doublethink in order to see the contradictory good and the bad simultaneously, and that is definitely the case with McCormick and Sanger, the women behind the men behind the pill.

McCormick had considered training as a doctor when she graduated in 1904, but instead she was seduced by the charms of Stanley McCormick, the well-educated heir to the American Harvester fortune, and married him. But by 1906, Mr McCormick was hospitalised for a year with what appeared to be schizophrenia, and by 1909 he was declared legally incompetent, suffering from violent paranoid delusions, and was looked after thereafter by male nurses on his estate in Montecito, California. He was so violent that McCormick couldn't have contact with him, but she occasionally watched him on visits through binoculars.

Sad as this was, it left Mrs McCormick extremely rich, single and bored. (Perhaps if the McCormicks had had children, the sexual revolution would have come much later.) McCormick threw herself into campaigning for votes for women, financed a suffrage magazine, and by 1917 had met Margaret Sanger and joined the Committee of 100, a group of women who were promoting the legalisation of 'birth control', a new phrase invented by Sanger. She believed that 'enforced motherhood is the most complete denial of a woman's right to life and liberty', and was horrified by what she saw among women debilitated by constant childbearing and botched street abortions in the poorest communities in New York. 'No woman can call herself free who does not own and control her body. No woman can call herself free until she can choose consciously whether she will or will not be a mother.'

Meanwhile, Sanger set up the American Birth Control League in 1921 (which later became Planned Parenthood), but she was also a racist and eugenicist, and said that 'birth control is nothing more or less than the facilitation of the process of weeding out the unfit [and] of preventing the birth of defectives.'[2] She also believed that 'Knowledge of birth control is essentially moral. Its general, though prudent, practice must lead to a higher individuality and ultimately to a cleaner race.'[3] Acknowledging this racist and ableist history, in 2020 Planned Parenthood in New York disavowed Sanger and her 'harmful connections to the eugenics movement' and removed her name from the clinic.[4] McCormick, however, gets a better write-up from Planned Parenthood, as a 'fierce feminist and secret smuggler'[5] who fought for the contraceptive cause for years.

In the 1920s, diaphragms (a rubber dome that fits into the vagina to prevent sperm reaching the cervix) were available in Europe but illegal to import into the US, where there was no manufacturer. Sanger wanted diaphragms, also known coyly as 'womb veils', for desperate women in New York. So, in an early foray into contraceptive provision in 1922, McCormick went on a grand European tour to cities like Rome and Paris, which happened to be home to the largest diaphragm manufacturers. Multilingual, she posed as a French or German scientist and ordered hundreds of diaphragms, which were delivered to her Swiss chateau. There, she had the diaphragms sewn into the silk lining of coats, or wrapped as presents, and took them back on an ocean liner to New York in eight steamer trunks, which easily passed through customs. Around a thousand diaphragms migrated from the silk-lined coats into the vaginas of Manhattan's poor, protecting them from procreation. McCormick also hid more diaphragms in cosmetics boxes sent into Canada, which were delivered to New York by alcohol smugglers during Prohibition. Eccentric as all this may seem, it reveals that McCormick would go to any lengths, legal or illegal, in her contraception crusade.

After her husband died in 1947, McCormick was free to spend his money however she wished. By the time Sanger introduced her to Dr Pincus at a New York dinner party, McCormick was already in her seventies and had no time to waste, so began pouring money and advice into his research. She moved from California to Boston to keep a closer eye on the work and complained about the freezing cold.

Her new friend Dr Pincus was not a mainstream scientist, having been sidelined by his alma mater, Harvard

University, after he produced the first test-tube rabbit in 1934, and enthused about in-vitro fertilisation. Aldous Huxley's novel *Brave New World* had just been published, featuring the fictional version of in-vitro human fertilisation, and the press referred to Dr Pincus as 'Dr Frankenstein'. The Frankenbunny experiment was considered bad enough, but in that anti-Semitic era, Harvard was not without other biases against the radical scientist; one historian said Dr Pincus was seen 'as a self-advertising Jew who published too soon and talked too much.'[6]

After failing to keep a post at Harvard, Dr Pincus set up his own Worcester Foundation for Experimental Biology in Massachusetts, which became ground zero for the contraceptive pill. He was joined by Dr Rock, a radical Catholic gynaecology professor, also from Harvard, who had previously set up a pioneering infertility clinic at the Free Hospital for Women in Massachusetts and was an expert in human as well as laboratory research. He had tested progestin injections previously on apparently infertile patients, hoping a few months' break from ovulation would improve their success. Of the eighty patients who had a break from ovulation, thirteen got pregnant once the treatment stopped. This became known as the 'Rock Rebound'[7]. Meanwhile, Dr Pincus had tested the new progestin injection on rabbits, which stopped them breeding, well, like rabbits, so between them the two scientists were ready for human trials of progestin birth control. But how would they conduct them, given the restrictions on contraception in the US and the laborious process for Food and Drug Administration (FDA) approval?

THE INSANE ASYLUM TESTS

McCormick's correspondence from the early 1950s shows just how deeply entrenched she was in the plans for testing the pill on women. In one disturbingly callous letter to Sanger, she asked: 'How can we get a "cage" of ovulation females to experiment with – this being our clinical bottleneck?' Later, the answer appeared: 'Upon my complaining vigorously to Dr Pincus about our lack of clinical wherewithal, he came back the next day with a plan to use patients at the Massachusetts State [Insane] Hospital.'[8]

The study went ahead. While the relatives of the mentally ill patients were told about the experiment, suggesting it would help with mood, the patients themselves did not give official consent. Dr Pincus administered the progestin injections to twelve female and – surprisingly – sixteen male psychiatric patients at Worcester State Hospital. He wanted to see whether the men's fertility was affected by progestin too, but the experiment foundered after one man's testicles shrank and the patients refused to give sperm samples.

The drug did seem to be stopping ovulating in the more compliant women, however. In further tests on his infertility patients, Dr Rock also used a twenty-day regime, which would prevent ovulation and still allow women to 'menstruate' (i.e. have a pill bleed during a week's break every month). With this change, Dr Rock thought the Catholic Church would be persuaded that progestin contraception was a 'natural' form of birth control.

These small sleight-of-hand experiments on the infertile

and the supposedly insane would never be approved as a proper clinical contraceptive trial by the FDA, so after considering experiments in Japan and Hawaii, the gang of four – Rock, Pincus, McCormick and Sanger – settled on Puerto Rico, an American territory with no birth control laws, as an ideal testing ground. In many ways, it functioned as an American colony. There was already a network of clinics, partly financed by the Americans, offering contraception and sterilisation. McCormick financed the final push in Puerto Rico, and was described by Elizabeth, Dr Pincus' wife, as a warrior: 'She carried herself like a ramrod. Little old woman she was not. She was a grenadier.'[9]

THE 'CONTRACEPTIVOS' TRIAL

In 1956, Dr Rock and Dr Pincus set up a clinic in San Juan, Puerto Rico, on what had previously been the worst, overpopulated slum on the island: the 'Little Mud Hole', or El Fangito. It was here that a new housing complex, Rio Piedras, had been built for the poor, with flats with running water and balconies. Many of the complex's residents had begun work for American companies on the island and were keen to raise their living standards and have smaller families. The offer of a contraceptive pill must have seemed a godsend to some in this Catholic country, although a few recruits were apparently students encouraged to join the experimental cohort to get better grades. Dr Pincus noted that '265 Puerto Rican housewives'[10] were enrolled into what they called the 'contraceptivos' trial.

One woman, known as Senora JG, was thirty years old and had ten children, aged ten months to sixteen years old. She also had a husband who 'drank heavily and insisted on daily intercourse but claimed to be too ill to work'.[11] Another woman had five children and a husband who was hospitalized frequently for mental illness. But the issue of informed consent remains – how on earth could it be informed? The whole experiment was deeply murky. The women of San Juan risked their health and lives in ways which have benefited millions worldwide who now take the pill. We should be putting up a plaque to those first pill-users. They were pioneers, but were treated as guinea pigs. Dr Rock wrote in his protocols that the women 'must be sufficiently intelligent to understand the general purpose of the experiment and their part in it.'[12] But while the women were told of the effects of the pill as birth control, they were given no information on risk or side effects, both of which were almost completely unpredictable.

Three young women died during the test phase, but the cause of their deaths was 'unknown' and never investigated. The propensity of the early pill, particularly in super-high doses, to cause blood clots and strokes was probably revealed here but not understood. What I can't understand is how these three deaths were dismissed in the final research presentations. But the fact is that one in ninety of those Puerto Rican women may have died trying out the first pill for us. 'How many of my fellow doctors are aware that the most popular method of contraception can be credited to medical experimentation on colonial subjects?'[13] wrote Dr Annabel Sowemimo in her book

Divided: Racism, medicine and why we need to decolonise health-care. 'We need to carefully examine the records of our institutions and not forget the colonial and racist practices which have become cemented as scientific knowledge.'[14]

The women of Rio Piedras (and later over a thousand more around the island) were given high doses of Searle's norethynodrel-estrogen tablet, Enovid, with no safety warnings. It was a contraceptive sledgehammer. The Enovid 10 pill contained 9.85mg of progestin, compared to present doses which are much, much smaller – between 0.1mg to 3mg. The pill also included 150mcg of a synthetic estrogen, mestranol. Nowadays the dose is between 20mcg and 50mcg of estrogen. Reports that 17 per cent of the women in the study had complained of nausea, dizziness, headaches, stomach pain and vomiting were not surprising – but they were dismissed.

Here, another unacknowledged woman pops up in the story: Dr Edris Rice-Wray, the American medical director of the Puerto Rico Family Planning Association, who was in charge of the trials on the ground. After a year, Dr Rice-Wray reported that the pill was 100 per cent effective when taken properly; one pregnancy had occurred, but the woman was considered to have failed to take the pill regularly. There was rejoicing at the success, but Dr Rice-Wray warned she had serious reservations. The patients' reactions were so severe and sustained that Dr Rice-Wray told Dr Pincus that the 10mg dose of Enovid caused 'too many side reactions to be generally acceptable.'[15] She was ignored, and the women were dismissed as 'unreliable historians'. Dr Pincus and Dr Rock thought their patients in Massachusetts had experienced far fewer negative reactions, and suggested the Puerto Ricans' complaints might be psychosomatic, despite clear evidence to the contrary. Dr Pincus did admit that in the first year of the trial that 25 per cent of the women quit 'because they either lost interest or found the medication undesirable'.[16] From the very start, women's voices around the pill were not listened to. The scientific patriarchy had very selective hearing.

The Enovid pill had only been properly tested on 130 women by the time Dr Pincus submitted his research to the FDA, but he masked the actual numbers by saying the pill had prevented pregnancy in 1,279 menstrual cycles, which sounded better, and the side effects were quietly sidelined. But what was the FDA doing allowing such sloppy research through? Standards were lower then, and a simple toxicity test was often all that was needed for some drugs. I also suppose the FDA had no idea how nuclear the pill's effect would be in terms of mass health or cultural change.

In 1957, Enovid was only approved at first for 'disorders of the female reproductive system' and not for general contraceptive use. The 1958 brochure on the contraceptive Enovid was not for patient education, but for medical professionals only, and it is in the Harvard archive. Under 'How Tolerated' the brochure lists: 'Nausea, although its reported incidence has varied widely, usually disappears on continuing treatment. Still less common side actions are vomiting and infrequently breast engorgement.'[17] Dizziness, headaches and even death seem to have conveniently disappeared from the list. Searle asked the FDA for approval of Enovid as a contraceptive a few years after, and by 1960 the pill was available throughout the country. The party had started. Within two years, 1.2 million American women were on it. Side effects be damned . . . for a while.

THE GREAT BRITISH PILL SCANDAL

Meanwhile, back in Blighty, clinical trials of the same pill, relabelled Conovid, began in 1960 in Birmingham, under the auspices of the Family Planning Association. Scientific rigour went to pot there, too. The pills were to cost 17 shillings a month, 15 shillings (roughly £15 now) of which would be paid by the NHS, so in a very British way the FPA charity thought it best to keep expenses down, and actually cut up the pills to give much lower doses of estrogen and only 2.5mg of progestin. That was good for side effects, but not for pregnancy. Of the forty-eight fertile women in the trial (all of whom had previously had a baby and had an 'average frequency of coitus not less than once weekly'[18]), a whacking fourteen got pregnant within three months. Disaster. But luckily the women of Slough came to the rescue. In that second trial, they were given 2.5mg of progestin, but topped up with higher levels of estrogen, and the combination seemed to work. Only one out of thirty-eight patients became pregnant, and the FPA medical officer said sniffily that 'could not be attributed to failure of the tablets, but to the patient's low IQ'.[19]

By 1961, after these tiny and questionable trials, the UK government decided the pill would be available on the NHS. Ironically, the MP who announced that women could have the pill, and ushered in sexual liberation, was the then Minister for Health, Enoch Powell. Seven years later he became infamous for his racist, anti-immigration 'Rivers of Blood' speech. As Powell pronounced the pill's debut in Parliament, a Labour MP asked: 'Is it left to the doctor to decide whether these pills shall be prescribed both for married and single women?' and Powell answered, rather radically: 'It is always for the individual doctor to decide in each case what are the medical requirements.'[20] In practice, only married women were really able to get the pill in the UK, until 1967 when family planning clinics were allowed to issue it to single women too. In 1962, only 50,000 British women were on the pill, but that rose to around one million in 1969. So, the Swinging Sixties swung rather later than you'd think in Britain.

THE POPE AND FAKE PERIODS

In the US, pill promotion continued apace. While Dr Pincus had done the scientific work (and doctored the results), Dr Rock took the crusade into the public eye. His book *The Time Has Come: A Catholic Doctor's Proposals to End the Battle over Birth Control* came out in 1963 and was covered by major news magazines and television. He was desperately keen to bring Catholics into the contraceptive fold, and for the Pope to approve of the pill within marriage. In his work as an obstetrician and gynaecologist, he had seen the physical and psychological horrors of non-stop childbearing, collapsed wombs and home abortions. So, Dr Rock tried to put the public case that using the pill was similar to using the rhythm method.

Previously, McCormick had been surprised to discover that Dr Rock was a practising Catholic and wrote in her letters: 'I was mistaken, and I learned recently that he does belong to the Catholic Church. How they put up with him I do not know!'[21] In one 1965 article in the *Massachusetts Patriot Ledger* newspaper, titled 'Catholic doctor urges planned parenthood', Dr Rock explains that the pill is artificial in a pharmaceutical sense but 'is natural in a physiological sense. It is not a foreign body once it gets into the feminine system.'[22] (Synthetic progestins are definitely foreign bodies, but Dr Rock perhaps genuinely thought otherwise.) He also claimed wrongly that the pill had no adverse relationship with cancer.

This was all part of the big sell, which included an attempt to make the pill look natural, with a monthly fake bleed when the synthetic hormones were withdrawn. This 'Pope Rule', as we now know, was unnecessary and put women through hormonal fluctuations, increased pregnancy risk, and kept sanitary towel manufacturers in profit. But the natural argument did not convince Pope Paul VI, and in 1968 the Church put out an encyclical *Humane Vitae* (on human life), giving the holy thumbs-up to the natural cycles of the rhythm method, and the thumbs-down to any artificial form of contraception. He condemned any 'act of mutual love which impairs the capacity to transmit life' and pointed out that contraception 'frustrates His design which constitutes the norm of marriage.'[23]

Dr Rock was heartily disappointed; later in life, he stopped attending church. His religious intervention, however, played on. For years, millions of women had millions of fake periods that were completely unnecessary. The FDA approved a three-month no-bleed pill in 2003, and a 365-day regime in 2007, and in the UK in 2000, the eminent gynaecologist Professor John Guillebaud said in *The Lancet* that monthly withdrawal bleeds were unnecessary.[24] Obviously, some women like to have a break, but the choice was never made clear. We did a survey in 2023 of 4,000 UK women for the *Pill Revolution* TV programme, and 48 per cent still thought you needed to bleed on the pill.

Unwittingly, Dr Rock, Dr Pincus, Sanger and McCormick unleashed a worldwide sexual revolution in the sixties, when their intention was to promote birth control and limit population growth. By 1965, 6.5 million American women were taking the pill daily, making it the most popular form of contraception, and it had begun to spread worldwide. Dr Pincus himself had always intended the use of the pill in a decent, upstanding marriage: 'I am against women having sexual freedom,' he in a 1967 interview. 'But I hasten to add that I am also opposed to sexual freedom among men.'[25] Dr Pincus was celebrated for his genius and in 1965 was elected to the National Academy of Sciences. After his death in 1967 from a bone marrow disease, ironically a side effect of long-term exposure to laboratory chemicals, he merited a huge obituary in the *New York Times* and elsewhere. In the same year, McCormick died, in Boston, at the ripe old age of ninety-two. There were no obituaries for her in any major papers.

THE FEMINIST BACKLASH

While early feminists like McCormick and Sanger fought for the pill, later feminists fought back against the patriarchal control of science. Reports from doctors of young women suddenly having blood clots after taking the pill began to appear within a few years of its launch. In 1969, the American investigative medical journalist Barbara Seaman published *The Doctor's Case Against the Pill*, gathering witness statements from women who had reported blood clots, strokes and other side effects including weight gain, decreased sex drive and depression while using the contraceptive, and interviews with doctors and researchers who questioned its safety. Seaman wrote later, 'Enovid was a chemical swamp, for, amid sworn assurances of safety, it began its commercial life as a massive overdose. Only after millions of women had taken Enovid – and thousands had died or had been disabled by blood clots – was it discovered that the amount of hormones in the pill was ten times what is needed for contraception.'[26] The unchecked power of the major pharmaceutical companies and the FDA's collusion came into question. Seaman's book alerted Democrat Senator Gaylord Nelson, who was investigating the pharmaceutical industry, and he managed to arrange a Senate hearing into the risks of the birth control pill.

In January 1970, testimony began in the Senate committee from experts: obstetricians, gynaecologists and psychiatrists who had opposing opinions on the safety and usefulness of the pill. What they mostly had in common were that they were men. Dr Francis Kane, a psychiatrist at the University of North Carolina Medical School, testified that he had seen women become psychotic and even suicidal after having used the pill. The only woman to speak was Dr Elizabeth Connell, an obstetrician and gynaecologist at the Columbia College of Physicians and Surgeons, who was worried about women being frightened off the pill. 'These are that the pills are not suitable for all women – in fact may be harmful to some – but that oral contraceptives are extremely beneficial to large numbers of women who for various reasons are not able to effectively use other contraceptive methods,' she said, as reported in the *New York Times*. The newspaper described Dr Connell as a 'petite blonde mother of six who testified for 2½ hours'.[27]

In the Senate audience, a large group of women were livid that the testimony of female patients was not included in the evidence, and that their doctors had not informed them of the risks of the pill. Alice Wolfson, from the radical collective D.C. Women's Liberation, jumped up and asked why no women were testifying. She shouted, 'Why is there no pill for men?' and 'Why are 10 million women being used as guinea pigs?' She also questioned the testimony of drug companies that were damaging women for profit and convenience: 'Why have you told them that they could get top priority? They're not taking the pills, we are!'[28] Senator Nelson said that the hearings should not be interrupted: 'If you ladies would, ah . . . sit down . . . ' to which Wolfson answered, 'We are not going to sit quietly! We don't think the hearings are any more important than our lives.' Then she was removed by a security marshal.

Cue a media shitstorm, and growing attention for the inquiry which was making the nightly television news.

In America, an estimated 87 per cent of women aged twenty-one to forty-five followed the hearings, and 18 per cent stopped taking the pill as a result.[29] In an interview in 2021,[30] Wolfson said: 'Remember, we were never against the pill. What we were against was a lack of informed consent. But from there, one of our questions was, "Now, why is there so much opposition to just telling a woman what could happen on the pill?"' The women started a sit-in at the Health Secretary's office to demand a warning on the birth control pill packet. 'That's what we were asking for. Not take the pill off the market; give us a warning. Tell us what's going to happen.' After much faffing around, the FDA eventually put a hundred-word warning on pill packets, which mentioned clot risk and danger signals like coughing up blood or swollen legs. Later, the hormone levels in the pill were brought down to lower doses and a patient information sheet was created for pharmaceuticals.

After the hearings, Wolfson worked with Seaman to build the campaigning National Women's Health Network. They were aware of their debt to the first women who took the pill, from Puerto Rico onwards. Seaman summed it up: 'I still frequently think about those women of an earlier generation who took the first pill – unaware of their part in a still unfolding experiment – and died for love.'[31] While the advent of the pill eventually brought unprecedented equality, educational opportunities, freedom of choice, and plenty of sex to more than 150 million women and counting, the drug's history is also repulsively mired in exploitation, colonisation, misogyny and racism. Thanks to a feminist philanthropist, a family-planning eugenicist and two male scientists who fudged their results and dismissed patients' health risks, millions more women went to university, and millions more flourished in their jobs. The pill was a giant step forward for the women's rights movement, but it was a step taken on the backs of the mentally ill, the poor and the disenfranchised. From the very beginning, women on hormonal contraception were never informed as consumers about what they were putting into their bodies. That's not entirely changed.

CHAPTER THIRTEEN

MALE CONTRACEPTION

Every unplanned pregnancy has a penis behind it, so why have women carried the burden of contraception for so long? Why have women been the ones using synthetic hormones on their bodies for the last sixty years? Why can't we share the joy of sex, and the responsibility too? The world of male contraception has recently leapt into the future after being stuck in the doldrums of the condom for years. Awaiting official approval, there are thrilling developments including a rub-on contraceptive shoulder gel; a temporary, meltable jelly vasectomy; a sperm discombobulator; a pill and a testicle-taming bath, more of which later.

RESPONSIBLE EJACULATIONS

As gender bias is questioned in every area of life, people are now talking about a moral imperative for men (and other people possessing penises) towards 'responsible ejaculations'. Dr Arianne Shahvisi, a senior lecturer in ethics at Brighton Medical School, led the charge on responsible ejaculating in the *British Journal of Medical Ethics*: 'I argue that men should take primary responsibility for protecting against pregnancy. Male long-acting reversible contraceptives are currently in development, and, once approved, should be used as the standard method for avoiding pregnancy. Since women assume the risk of pregnancy when they engage in penis-in-vagina sex, men should do their utmost to ensure that their ejaculations are responsible, otherwise women shoulder a double burden of pregnancy risk plus contraceptive responsibility.'[1] No longer should women be irresponsibly 'knocked up' before ending up 'up the duff', with 'a bun in the oven' while 'eating for two' and 'harbouring a fugitive'. It's a shared liability now.

Dr Shahvisi also wrote another essay comparing contraceptive justice and the way society expected us to behave during the Coronavirus epidemic. Wearing a condom to protect a woman from the health risk of pregnancy is similar to wearing a mask to avoid infecting the old and vulnerable with Covid-19. 'Instead of thinking of women as being vulnerable to pregnancy, we should think of men as carrying serious risks that they must act to minimise.' Dr Shahvisi also points out that contraception is burdensome for women because it's costly, and the associated medical appointments take time and planning, and can be uncomfortable. 'Most forms of contraception also come with serious side effects, and abortions can be medically serious and are still widely stigmatised. These costs are particularly morally concerning because they're sex-asymmetric.'[2]

For centuries, men have confidently offered the withdrawal method as contraception, and minutes later apologised profusely when it went wrong – that's about a fifth of the time, according to Planned Parenthood.[3] Will women trust men to remember to rub a contraceptive gel on their shoulder every morning? Will they believe a man when says he has a temporary gel vasectomy? There is a different level of trust and honesty between most couples, but out there in the bedroom rodeo of Tinder and Bumble, among strangers who are hooking up rather than settling down, can women – who bear the risk – take a gamble on men's truth? Probably not. (We all know everyone should be using condoms to start with, in case of sexually transmitted diseases, but we also know that's not a reflection of reality.)

Attitudes among couples are different. In a survey of almost two thousand women attending family planning clinics across Scotland, China and South Africa, 65 per cent thought that the responsibility for contraception falls too much on women. Only 13 per cent of the total sample did not think that hormonal male contraception was a good idea and only 2 per cent said that they would not trust their partner to use it.[4] On TikTok, there are dozens of videos vox-popping men about their attitudes, but a more scientific take comes from a paper by Professor Richard Anderson at the University of Edinburgh, one of the experts behind the male contraceptive shoulder gel, which we will detail later.[5] They analysed thirty-two studies and found that in new drug trials, between 34 and 82 per cent of men were willing to use a male contraceptive, and for women, between 43 and 94 per cent were happy for their partner to try it. Younger men were more open to male contraception than older ones.[6] There's a changing desire out there to share responsibility, and a desire for safer contraception.

MEN WANT AGENCY IN CONTRACEPTION TOO

Politics is also a massive part of this new picture. As abortion rights are ripped away in countries from America to Poland, there's been a rethink, particularly among men, about their right not to have a baby by mistake. Plus, in a post #MeToo world, a place where gender equality matters more, many men want to share responsibility for conception, which could be the most important event in their lives. As barriers fall, and gender becomes more fluid, improving male contraception also empowers many transgender women, non-binary and intersex people too.

L.R. Fox, the CEO of NEXT Life Sciences, which is making the Plan A contraceptive, which uses the new reversible Vasalgel vasectomy gel said: 'Long-acting reversible contraception is what men hope to see, and the holy grail is a non-hormonal version. Women can set and forget with the copper coil without having to use a devastating hormonal method. I'm also not sure if most women would fully trust their partner to apply a daily gel or pill – I can barely remember to take a multivitamin.' Fox wishes he had known about the future promise of Plan A when he

was younger. 'I've had my vasectomy and my decision to
have one stemmed from my experience as a child. I grew
up in the foster care system, seeing first-hand the devastating consequences that follow from parents not being
ready for their children.' This reversible choice for men is
needed more than ever – in the months after the Roe v.
Wade decision was overturned in America, vasectomies
increased by 30 per cent, and as much as 39 per cent in
states that had completely banned abortion.[7]

'It's not about shifting the burden, it's about alleviating
the burden that's been largely carried by women for far
too long. We need to share responsibility, each making
intentional decisions, so we need options that allow men
to take action and participate in contraception,' said Fox.
Perhaps because Fox originally comes from outside the
world of medicine, he thinks a bit more outside the box.
'We still live in a world which denies us when exactly
we choose to have a child, with the main option being to
just pump women full of hormones,' – unless you wear a
condom. 'Imagine this being taught in a history class in the
future. Kids would ask, "Were previous people just idiots
or did you just hate women? You couldn't plan the most
important decision of your life, and you called yourselves
advanced?"'

Apart from the vasectomy, the withdrawal method
and the condom, there have been no other options for
men – until now. Rubber condoms were first produced
in 1855, although for centuries people with penises had
resorted to all sorts of protective business with animal
intestines, or linen and string. In 1932, the London Rubber

Company produced the lighter and more flexible latex Durex condom. Yet despite over a century of use, the patriarchy often panics when faced with a prophylactic in a darkened room. And as comedian Kathy Lette said: 'Many fellas think riding bareback makes them more of a stallion.' Condom use is down among young people[8] and among divorced retirees who are getting back in the sack. One consultant at an NHS sexual health clinic in London admitted to me, 'No one ever comes in and asks us for a condom nowadays.'

In one (apparently serious) academic study, men were given an astonishing forty-six different reasons to choose from on why they would, or would not, wear a condom. The culprits included the usual 'reduces sensation', 'ruins foreplay', 'destroys romance', 'doesn't fit right', 'we were drunk', 'God told me not to' and even 'I'm too well endowed'. Of course, many women hate condoms too, for the discomfort, embarrassment and increased risk. In a small Hanx condom survey, over half of UK lovers said they had gone ahead and had unprotected sex because they didn't want to discuss using a condom.[9]

But with sexually transmitted diseases like gonorrhoea and chlamydia – and even old-fashioned ones like syphilis – now making a huge comeback in Britain and the US[10] [11], barrier methods are a no-brainer. Then there is also the grim practice of 'stealthing': taking off a condom during sex, putting the other person at risk of STDs or pregnancy. In 2021, a British man was convicted of rape after he purposely took off a condom, although he had agreed with the sex worker beforehand to wear one.[12] Dr Tara Suchak, who

specialises in HIV sexual health, says the availability of the
HIV-prevention drug PReP has made people less obsessed
with using condoms, and they know most STDs can be
treated, although there are often long waits for clinics.
But let's be straightforward: in consensual sex, if you feel
you can't ask a man to use a condom for the first time, he
probably shouldn't be in your bed.

In the UK, we use 3 million condoms a week, and in
the US, it's over 8 million. For gentlemen who still want
'Something for the weekend, sir?' – a euphemism from
when condoms were sold in barbers' shops – things have
very much improved, not just in terms of vegan latex,
'longer-lasting' lubricant, ribbing, dots or a glow-in-
the-dark option. Roam condoms come in more inclusive
skin tones, like dark brown and light brown, and there's
a smorgasbord of sizes available from one international
manufacturer, MyOne, with ten lengths and ten circum-
ferences to choose from. Customers can calculate their
own size by downloading a measuring kit off the website.
Durex also has a similar 'FitFinder Tool' online; basically you print off a small paper measuring tape, wrap it
round your penis, and work out whether you want Close,
Regular or Wide.

This twenty-first-century resizing makes more sense,
as industry regulators originally declared condoms should
be 7.3 inches, to ensure maxi coverage, but for most men
that's far too long and bunches up uncomfortably at the
bottom of the shaft. It turns out that a review of erect
penis sizes around the world (who wanders around with a
ruler doing this sterling work?) revealed that the average

was 5.2 inches, and a US study varied between 1.6 inches and 10.2 inches.[13] Good to know.

Reading the various condom websites, I also realised that many of us lack basic condom-launching skills, which were never taught to us by the sex-ed teacher with the banana. The how-to advice says: first up, check the sell-by date. Second, shoogle the condom to one side in the packet so you don't rip it on opening, and don't use sharp items like your teeth. Hanx biodegradable condoms advise pinching the top of the condom between thumb and forefinger to get rid of trapped air, which could make the condom split during action. The tip is where the semen will go. Roll the condom on from the top down. The website adds: 'When it's all over, keep hold of the condom at the base of the penis to make sure it doesn't slip off while you pull out. Take the condom off, tie a knot in it (no balloon animals, we beg you) so that the contents don't spill out and wrap it in a tissue.' They suggest eco-composting afterwards.

MALE HORMONAL CONTRACEPTION

Moving on from the condom, the story continues in the 1950s in the Wild West of clinical trials with equally unpleasant experimentation on men and women. Dr John Rock, the American who pushed through the mass female pill trials in Puerto Rico, did some early unethical experiments in 1954 testing an oral progestin contraceptive on twelve female and sixteen male psychiatric patients at Worcester State Hospital in Massachusetts, an asylum that burned down in 1991. The patients were given the high doses of hormones without their consent, although Professor Rock said he did inform next of kin, but he claimed he was testing the tranquillising effect of the drugs. I can't find any record of what the women said, but the men complained of serious side effects: the pill was giving them feminine characteristics, shrinking their testicles and their voices were changing. They refused to give sperm samples, and the experiment was shut down.

Previously, researchers had found that giving men injections of testosterone could lower sperm counts; the testes stopped production as testosterone was pumped into the brain and body from elsewhere. Studies using testosterone alone showed that the method was successful with few adverse effects but adding a progestin increased suppression of millions of sperm more quickly and effectively. Once the progestin and testosterone were present together in the injections, men complained of side effects like acne, injection site pain, mood change, lowered or increased libido and weight gain. Those side effects may seem very familiar on a daily basis to women on the pill now, but they were considered severe enough to leave the male pill in research limbo for years.

Moving on to the 1980s, researchers tried blocking a different hormone, gonadotropin-releasing hormone (GnRH), which controls the production of hormones necessary for sperm production. (Some women who have endometriosis are given GnRH blockers to put them into temporary menopause to shut down estrogen production, which can worsen the condition.) Monthly injections of the GnRH hormone started in men, but – guess what? – the method was associated with significant side effects, including depression and decreased bone density. So, another male contraceptive bit the dust. Are there more double standards here? We still give women the Depo-Provera injection, which can cause a fall in bone density. The Royal Osteoporosis Society says Depo-Provera can increase your risk of osteoporosis and broken bones. 'This mainly happens in the first few years on Depo-Provera, then the bone density stabilizes,' they said on their website. That's still not reassuring.

Until recently, efforts to create gender equality on the contraceptive front have been pretty pathetic, and certainly not at the top of the multinational pharmaceutical companies' wish list. We already have cheap baby-blocking in generic contraceptive pills for women, so Big Pharma does not want to risk billions in trials of risky new male options. Thus it has been mostly left to governments and academic institutions to stand courageously between the sperm and the egg. But even the World Health Organization (WHO) had cold feet when it came to hormonal contraception for men. A testosterone and progestin injection trial was suddenly cancelled in 2016 despite successful sperm suppression and a pregnancy rate of 1.5 per cent (better than the female pill). But a minority suffered side effects, some of which included acne, mood swings and even increased libido. This provided months of entertainment for feminists — 'Big boys can't handle teensy weensy side effects!' — but took us no further forward.

The WHO Human Reproduction Program Research Project Review Panel also said: 'The frequencies of mild to moderate mood disorders were relatively high.' While this is a regular problem for women on the pill, it turns out that in male contraception trials, side effects are given more scientific weight because a man cannot get pregnant. Female contraceptive risk is weighed against the risks of, say, blood clots or even death in pregnancy. The Male Contraceptive Initiative charity is trying to get this bias changed, so men can be part of the 'shared risk' as a couple. Right now, a male contraceptive has to be of a higher standard of tolerability than a female one.

THE BRAVE NEW WORLD OF MALE CONTRACEPTION

But there is, at last, growing excitement in the scientific world around contraceptive development, among mice and men. It's hard to tell what is the most promising, and some have not yet reached human trials, but there's an amazing choice out there, much of it non-hormonal. A non-hormonal male contraceptive (known boringly as YCT529, rather than Taking the Mickey) prevents pregnancy in mice by blocking a vitamin A receptor, with no obvious side effects. It dramatically reduced sperm counts in male mice over four weeks and was 99 per cent effective in preventing pregnancy. Plus, the mice fathered babies again just over a month after they stopped contraception.[14] Trials began on sixteen British men in 2023.

The assault on sperm is taking many routes. Like tadpoles, sperm need to waggle their tails (or flagella) asymmetrically to navigate towards the egg, and at Yale

School of Medicine in the US, cell biologist and associate professor Jean-Ju Chung says that if sperm are able to swim only in straight lines they will lose the ability to navigate. So she is targeting a protein in the sperm tail and editing out the gene in animal models. Watch this space for humans.

Over at Weill Cornell Medicine in New York, Professors Jochen Buck and Lonny Levin are working on an on-demand contraceptive that stops fertility almost immediately. Their compound could be a pill, but it is presently an injection being tested in mice, and it would stop sperm from swimming altogether, so long as it was taken around thirty minutes before sex, and it would probably have effects that last until the morning after. Their research is still ongoing and is being supported by the Male Contraception Initiative.

At last, there seems to be a flurry of ballsy innovation, both hormonal and non-hormonal, in this space. In Germany, Rebecca Weiss won a Dyson award in 2021 for her plans for an ultrasound mini-bath for the testicles, which involved using ultrasound deep heat for a few minutes, temporarily halting sperm mobility so they can no longer fertilise an egg. After the bath, the process takes two weeks to work, and then needs to be topped up every few months to keep the sperm ineffective, but does not suppress blood testosterone levels. Photographs show the COSO, a stylish mini-bath device Apple would be proud of in orange, grey or black, which after an initial test can eventually be used at home. It was brilliantly described by the *New York Post* as 'A Sperm-Stopping Sauna for the

Scrotum' and has also provided hours of TikTok fun. The COSO is now heading into the clinical testing phase. Men I've discussed this option with seem a tad nervous, but confidence may grow in time.

But while we wait for the science to go through human trials, vasectomy remains the only option left for men who don't want risks or condoms. I chatted to a friend over tea about his vasectomy. His memories were mildly traumatic rather than fond. 'I had to shave my balls! Then a nurse came at me with a huge needle and injected each testicle. Supposed to anaesthetise it, but it was bloody sore. And then they got the scalpel,' he put down his mug, gesturing graphically, 'and made two cuts, and then they went in and closed off the tubes and put in some stitches. It was painful for at least a week, longer till I recovered completely.' But my friend does have a large number of offspring, and he's pleased he did it.

That was a few years ago, and now the newer no-scalpel vasectomy is being rolled out privately and in the NHS. It works by making a tiny hole in the scrotum and heals more quickly. About 20 per cent of men in the UK get a vasectomy, and 10 per cent in the US, but that's on the rise and there are long waiting lists since the abortion laws changed in 2022. Planned Parenthood recently offered free vasectomies in one state and was inundated with applicants within hours. But vasectomies are difficult to reverse and a mite scary, so it's not surprising that uptake is still low.

The temporary gel vasectomy

Fortunately, the temporary gel vasectomy, technically known as vasocclusion, is on the cards, and likely to go into human trials in with Plan A's Vasalgel the US soon. In Australia, the first twenty-five couples are already testing out the efficacy of a similar gel — almost inevitably called ADAM — in a three-year trial. Vasalgel is a hormone-free Long-Acting Reversible Contraception (LARC), a hydrogel which can be injected into the vas deferens, the tubes that carry the sperm out of the testes. Unlike a lifelong vasectomy, a few years later if the man wants to reverse the process, the sperm-blocking hydrogel can be dissolved away. Basically, it's a LARC for men who want to have larks, responsibly. Entrepreneur L.R. Fox, mentioned above, is the bearded twenty-something behind the Plan A trials in America, and he has also worked in the counterdrone industry. Previously his job was to 'detect pilotless aircraft in your vicinity . . . and keep your airspace safe.' It seems perfect that he is now keeping women safe from rogue sperm.

I got on a Zoom call with Fox to investigate. Fifty thousand people have signed up to hear more about the Vasalgel research, and the whole sperm-blocking package will be sold as Plan A. Is that name riffing off the fact the American morning-after pill brand is Plan B, I asked him. 'I can't confirm or deny that,' he said, laughing. 'We need to make important choices when we decide to have a child. It should be Plan A, not Plan B.'

Fox explained that Plan A refers to the whole package,

and we got technical: 'It starts with a lumen access [tube opening] device to hold the vas deferens in place on each side, because it's mobile, a bit like spaghetti. Then Vasalgel would be injected into the vas, and after delivery, this little bit of hydrogel forms a flexible filter within the body that is designed to block sperm.' Sort of a sieve blocking sperm? 'That's right. Because fluid, but not sperm, can flow through the filter that will avoid post-vasectomy pain that usually comes from back-up pressure. With Plan A, we intend to let all of the juice to pass through, with none of the seed.' The body doesn't just make sperm and store it — it keeps constantly recycling it. If sperm is not ejaculated, the cells die every couple of months and are reabsorbed into the body. Fox gave me the big sell: 'Our mission is to provide a ten-minute pain-free procedure, with ten years thought-free protection.' Actually, I imagine that the clamp and the injection might hurt a bit, but perhaps not so much as getting a coil inserted . . .

But what of the unblocking of the tubes, two, four, six, eight or ten years later when you want to have children? 'We dissolve the hardened gel with sodium bicarbonate solution.' Um, is that baking soda? 'Correct! Yes, the gel liquefies and flows out, and you clear your pipes. We won't ask about how you clear your pipes. But the intent is that after you've cleared and done a sperm test, you're ready to go!' Fox laughed. He wouldn't be drawn on the cost, but said they are working to ensure Plan A is as affordable and accessible as possible. 'We're not designing it to need a highly specialized doctor, but to be done by a wide variety of clinic staff. We also want to consider storage humidity and transportation, so it can get to rural America or tropical locations without any shelf-life issues.'

It's interesting – and disturbing – how much contraception innovation took place in countries where medical trials were less stringently regulated: Puerto Rico for the female pill, and India where the precursor to Vasalgel has been in development for decades. In India, Dr Sujoy K. Guha engineered a pump which filtered dirty water using a hydrogel lining inside pipes, which was polarised to deactivate bacteria. He moved on to creating a similar gel filter for male human pipes eventually called Reversible Inhibition of Sperm Under Guidance (RISUG). This Indian research reached phase three trials in men, a thirteen-year safety study which was 98 to 99 per cent effective, a good prevention rate, but the research was slowed by insufficient numbers of volunteers. 'They also discovered in interviews afterwards that some cases of pregnancy were caused by infidelity,' added Fox. The RISUG technology was then brought over to the United States by the not-for-profit Parsemus Foundation, developed into Vasalgel, and then tested on monkeys and baboons. 'These primate studies supported the product's safety, and contraception was effective,' said Fox. 'Males don't have a mating season, they're just at it all the time like us. It was the best animal trial to be in – two years of joyous fun and no babies.'

Now NEXT Life Sciences have to make the final push to get to market, and have labs 'working day and night' in California and Arizona, said Fox. 'We're looking forward to the start of our human trials to demonstrate the safety and effectiveness of Plan A to the FDA [Food and Drug

Administration].' Fox is hopeful, following clinical trials and a rapid FDA marketing authorisation, that it will be available in 2026.

How about a rub-on male contraceptive gel?

In Edinburgh, Professor Anderson has been working for the last few years on the UK arm of a worldwide trial, started by the US government-funded National Institutes of Health, of a male contraceptive gel made from testosterone and the progestin Nestorone. This NES/T (Nestorone/testosterone) Phase 2 study started in 2018 and ends in late 2024. Scientists recruited over four hundred couples across four continents, in cities including Edinburgh, Manchester, Los Angeles, Seattle, Nairobi and Santiago. The men rub the gel on their shoulders every morning, and eventually their sperm count goes from a normal full-throttle 40–200 million per millilitres down to below 1 million or even zero. I learned two useful words researching this: oligozoo-spermia, which means you have a low sperm count, less than 15 million sperm per millilitre, and azoospermia, which indicates none at all. The zoo is indeed empty.

After around three months of gel application and checks as the sperm count goes down, temporary azoospermia is usually achieved, and men are then pronounced ready for action. 'Obviously there aren't any official results out yet because there's still some way to go, since the final couples are now close to the end, but it certainly looks very encouraging,' said Professor Anderson. 'We're looking at something that will be as good as highly effective hormonal methods like the pill. In the order of a couple of percent of pregnancies per 100 women.' What happens if men miss a day's gel? 'Certainly erratic use of NES/T doesn't work, although the odd missed day is probably ok – as it is with the pill, unless it's at the beginning of a packet, so maybe not so different!'

Professor Anderson explains that the progestin component does most of the suppressing and switches off the sperm production. 'Then you need to give testosterone back, basically as HRT [hormone replacement therapy] because the testes are no longer producing it.' So there is very little testosterone in the testes, but plenty circulating in the rest of the body and the brain. 'It's just like the female pill suppressing ovulation. Nestorone is an up-and-coming progestin. It's very selective, and doesn't cause high blood pressure, or those clogging, clotting effects. But it's also extremely potent. You can't take it orally.' (I wondered whether Nestorone would be great for all sorts of female contraceptives too, and so far it is perfoming well in trials, according to the Population Council, in the form of a contraceptive vaginal ring. More on this in Chapter 14.) Plus the testosterone is body-identical and transdermal, whereas the old synthetic testosterone pills were damaging to the liver.

The only problem is that, for a few men, the sperm doesn't suppress to low enough levels to avoid pregnancy, but the checks over three months will show that. 'When the sperm count goes below one million, the men get the green light and they are good to go. The number of people who haven't suppressed is very, very small. And that may be to do with erratic use, or the different way people absorb it through the skin.' On side effects, Professor Anderson said: 'You can't get something for nothing. You have to change things to suppress sperm and inevitably some people will feel a bit different. But as I said, we're very hopeful.' It's only been thirty years of work for Professor Anderson. 'My wife keeps saying: "How come you've been doing this for so long and you still haven't got it right?"' He sighs again. The Phase 3 trials have yet to come, and he may well be retired by then. It could take five more years. 'We haven't got a huge pharmaceutical company behind this, writing million-dollar cheques. This is the NIH [National Institutes of Health] and cash is constantly a struggle for them, you know, constantly needing to renew their budgets every year and make sure they've got enough to keep the trial going.'

In an article in *Chemical and Engineering News* (not a publication I'd ever expected to consult), there was an interview with 28-year-old Alex Springer, who works in a biotech company in Seattle, and had signed up for the NES/T contraceptive trial. One of the reasons was because his partner Mel Hopkins, also twenty-eight, has type 1 diabetes and had struggled to control her blood sugar levels for years on hormonal contraception. She wanted a break. 'I think the onus is really on men to start to take a little bit more responsibility for family planning and contraceptive use,' said Springer. Every morning, after his shower, he pumps a squirt of gel into his hands and rubs it on both shoulders, and it dries in about thirty seconds. 'It just kind of becomes part of the routine,' he said.

The trial has checks in place for mental health, and reports so far say side effects have been minimal. I had a trawl round Reddit for anonymous user stories, and this one popped up. 'Tomorrow is my last day taking birth control for a clinical trial I have been participating in. I have enjoyed every second of the process and my girl-friend and I are gutted to be ending it. To summarise the side effects I have experienced: increased libido (has remained the same since I started the trial), much higher general energy levels, some low-level mood swings, weight gain (wait for the next point before reading into this too much), quite significant changes in my muscula-ture (hard to chalk up to just the birth control), increased irritability and aggression at times (don't worry, I haven't been knocking heads together in bar fights!).'

The Reddit writer added some useful caveats: he found his mood was best when he regularly used the gel in the morning, rather than at different times of day, and the weight gain was mostly muscle mass after signing up to a gym, so he had no idea whether the testosterone or exer-cise was the key. 'I think for me, the control I was able to have over my own fertility felt incredibly empowering and it is something I will miss dearly. Reproductive equality is missing from sex, and I think trials like these are SO important.'

THE STORY OF DAN, EMILY AND THEIR BABY SON JACK

I met Dan and Emily Glastonbury, who are both in their early thirties, and their one-year-old son Jack, at their house in Manchester. They were really welcoming and wanted to tell their story as a couple tackling male contraception. Their house is full of photographs of the family in pirate and other costumes – Dan is a children's entertainer – and piles of kids' picture books, batik hangings and sequinned cushions. Dan went on the Nestorone/testosterone gel trial back in April 2019, and was told he was 'safe to go' in June 2019. He successfully stayed on the gel until October 2020, and felt a bit bereft when the trial ended. It was Emily who originally found out about the scheme. 'I saw an advert on Facebook and I signed up without telling Dan at first. Women have handled it for such a long time, and I'd heard about the failed contraceptive trials for men, and it just all just seemed a bit unfair, really. It all felt like things needed to start changing. So, I thought, why not? Let's find out some more information and see where that takes us.' After a couple of drinks one evening, Emily told Dan what she'd done. He thought for a moment and then said: 'Why not?'

Dan explained: 'Looking at a list of the side effects a woman can have from the pill blew my mind, because every girl I knew was on some form of hormonal contraception. And it never occurred to me that there are so many things that women deal with on a day-by-day basis. Silently, you know, they just deal with it. Whereas if a man is presented with that same list of side effects, there's no way he would touch it. So, agreeing to the trial seemed to me to be helping progress towards some form of equality.' Plus, at the age of nineteen, Dan was hit by cancer and recovered after a tough year of chemo and radiation. He wrote a bucket list and the time, one entry was 'take part in a clinical trial'. He wanted to give something back. And it went well. 'I had no side effects, not a single one. I've a very physical job. I'm a children's entertainer and I throw kids up in air all the time and things like that. And in no way did I feel like weaker or slower or anything like that.'

Emily had never had an easy time with contraception, so that was an added incentive. When she first went on the pill as a teenager, her mother noticed it wasn't really agreeing with her and encouraged her to go back to the clinic and ask for a different pill. 'It took quite a while, nearly a year, trialling out lots of different ones to get on to one that was right for me. But I know lots of people don't have that, they don't know what's going on. And because you're still a teenager, you just think it's all part of being a teenager. You don't realise how much these things are affecting you.' More recently, she has had the hormonal coil for five years, and still remembers the agony of the fitting: 'I just remember it being so horribly painful that I saw colour emerge before my eyes and I didn't know whether it was normal or not. Nobody had really talked it through with me. Nobody had really gone into all of the ins and outs.'

Together, Dan and Emily decided it was his turn for contraception. But were they worried about Dan's fertility coming back afterwards? They laugh and point to Jack sitting on Emily's knee. He was conceived three months after the trial ended, when Dan's sperm count slowly came back to normal. But Dan did have some doubts at the start, as his sperm count went down from 42 million to lower than a million. 'It's lowering your sperm count, purposely causing your body to become infertile. It's kind of scary that it might not come back. You know they said they can't a hundred per cent promise anything, but they are 99 per cent sure that it will be fine. So, there was this chance that we might not be able to have children. But as you can see . . . '

For Emily, giving up synthetic hormones gave her a chance to get in tune with her menstrual cycle for the first time in years. 'I began to be able to track things a bit better and notice lots of different changes within me. I had no idea what my body's natural rhythm was. So, it was great to get in touch with that. When you stop contraception, it's kind of crazy. It's almost like suddenly you realise it's like a light switching on.'

'The clouds lifting?' said Dan. Emily nods.

We discuss whether the NES/T gel would work for couples just dating rather than in a serious relationship. Dan says he tested the waters when he went on a stag do just after he started the trial. 'All my male friends were joking, "Don't touch me. I don't want to go infertile." So, there's that kind of thing around it. And lots of people say, you know, I'd never trust a man to take a contraception. I think there's that kind of sort of vibe about it. I think you need to be in a long-term relationship.'

If approved by regulatory authorities, in Phase 3 trials, the Nestorone/testosterone gel would be the first-of-its-kind contraceptive for men — more likely for men of Jack's generation than Dan's at this rate of progress. But Emily said they were just grateful to have been on the trial. 'It's been amazing. I think it definitely came along at a time in our lives where I really needed to have a break from the pill.'

They agree that having the man literally shoulder responsibility for contraception felt like an act of love. 'I think it brought us together closer as a couple as well,' said Dan.

Men's enthusiasm for potential solutions like Vasalgel temporary vasectomies and the NES/T shoulder gel contraceptive is clear, so why is it all taking so long? Professor Anderson sighed as he explained this, yet again: 'The problem with contraception is that it's just not a big money-spinner for the pharmaceutical companies. It's very much a bulk product for companies with very little profit margin and essentially, it's a product that has to work perfectly with zero side effects, which it does not. So it's not like saving people dying of cancer, where patients will put up with any side effects.'

In the three years leading up to 2021, only 11 per cent of global research and development budgets went on male contraception, compared to 71 per cent to female (the rest was unspecified). 'Contraception is a low-cost, very high-risk medication for companies to be involved in. That's why we have to get funding, very slowly, from elsewhere.' Most pharmaceutical companies are not benevolent, and research and development must equal profit. Capitalism controls contraception and is happy to continue selling the tried-and-tested, cheap-as-chips female pill. Yet there are estimates that the male contraception market could be worth up to $200 billion worldwide. Men genuinely want to share the contraceptive burden, and perhaps that cultural shift will speed up medical progress at last.

CHAPTER FOURTEEN

TAKING POWER OVER PLEASURE

In the end, this book is about us taking power over pleasure, getting a handle on our hormones, and having fantastic, fearless sex. This is why I'm filling this final chapter with good news about the future and the ways we can go forward as feminists, armed with science and self-knowledge, to demand the reproductive justice we deserve. I know *Everything You Need to Know About the Pill* is a pretty tough read at times. It was hard to write too, but I found that the bursts of anger every time I unearthed something really appalling just kept me going.

This is not just a story about contraception. It is a story of over half a century of neglect, dismissal and manipulation of women and their health, in which the patriarchy and Big Pharma play a dastardly role. There is also something more subtle going on: a paternalism – or perhaps maternalism – among the many brilliant institutions, health professionals and charities that provide contraceptive care, which results in a downplaying of risks and side effects. For those institutions, the greater good of keeping as many women and people with ovaries on contraception as possible is constantly being weighed against telling us the whole truth about what we are putting into our bodies.

We know very well that family planning increases education opportunities, reduces gender inequalities, improves child and maternal health, and through all that decreases poverty and hunger. But while health professionals talk about the wonderfully wide choice of contraceptives, most of those choices contain the usual suspects — synthetic progestins. It's time to move on, to question every medical and cultural orthodoxy, take the best from the past, look ahead at better forms of contraception — and develop a better understanding of our natural cycles and what hormones do in our brains.

BREAKING THE SILENCE

Across the world — from the Scandi academics investigating mental health to the Indian and American dream of the jelly vasectomy, and the British pharmacists exploring body-identical hormones — there are great scientific brains on the case. Thanks to the rise of female leaders in FemTech, Gen Z and Millennials at last have The Knowledge, accurate contraceptive information in apps like Clue and The Lowdown, public discussion on social media of conditions like PMS and endometriosis, and an understanding of the menstrual cycle in all its vagaries. Women are realising they are consumers with choices, and not just docile pill-poppers. Even in America, where abortion rights have been taken from women in twenty-four states, pills in the post have circumvented the law, and in states without bans, the abortion pill is increasingly available from pharmacies.

Plus, there's a growing conversation, the hive mind here and on TikTok and Instagram, and while that can sometimes be bonkers or inaccurate, it definitely gives us a voice. Or as @Traynor_swift put it on my @pills-candal Instagram account: 'I feel we need to investigate new forms of contraceptives. Women were led to believe the pill represented the sexual revolution – what piffle. We have been chemically castrated, so blokes get a shag without worry.' That's perhaps an exaggeration, but if 45 per cent of pregnancies are still unintended after all these years, then we most definitely need to question women's contentment with contraception and their access to it. The writer Audre Lorde, who described herself as 'a Black feminist lesbian poet warrior mother', said her decision to write honestly about her own health and breast cancer diagnosis was 'for other women of all ages, colors, and sexual identities who recognize that imposing silence about any areas of our life is a tool for separation and powerlessness.'[1] We are breaking that silence into a million little pieces.

At the same time, we need billions more spent on research. Until now, according to McKinsey, about 1 per cent of healthcare research – biopharma and med-tech – has been invested in female-specific conditions beyond oncology. You read that right: 1 per cent. 'Women account for 80 per cent of consumer purchasing decisions in the healthcare industry. Yet, remarkably, women's health has been considered a niche market and a mere subset of healthcare. Now, that's starting to shift,'² they reported. Investment in FemTech is growing, and *Forbes* magazine notes that 'women's healthcare is a market ripe for disruption and innovation'. They report that the large pharmaceutical companies, after years of recycling versions of much the same old products, are eyeing the next generation of companies in women's health, looking for innovation and providing venture capital. Like I said previously, capitalism has always driven contraception.

MAPPING OUR GENOMES AND HORMONES

But perhaps this time it's in our favour, as investment goes to young women and men who are thinking out of the box. When we made the *Pill Revolution* documentary, we went to visit Dama Health, a FemTech start-up in Cambridge, which has started mapping thousands of women's DNA so they can work out what hormones or pills suit each woman best, how strong their reactions are, and whether there are any intolerances. Basically, it's an ancestry.com-style test to give women information on what contraception will work best for them, and which one would involve the least side effects and risks, while also informing their likelihood of developing PMS, polycystic ovarian syndrome, blood clots, endometriosis and breast cancer. By taking medical histories, and comparing them with the genome, Dama will build up a picture of which biomarkers affect the interaction of contraception in women.

In among the white coats, glass labs, vast screens, banks of centrifuges and hipster break-out coffee areas, I met Elena Rueda Carrasco, the 28-year-old co-founder of Dama Health. She explained: 'Right now we very much have a trial-and-error prescribing process. There's no way of being able to anticipate side effects, or which concentrations of hormones are better suited to each women. Our work is therefore looking into the role of estrogen and progesterone genes, for example, and how women metabolize estrogen and progesterone – as we know this varies per person.' The genome-hormone mapping will eventually enable precision medicine, rather than patients being guinea pigs over and over. Like an ancestry test, you just need to send in a saliva sample from which they extract your DNA. Elena said: 'I was increasingly aware of women being gaslighted about their symptoms on hormonal contraception, and unheard. I want to get the data to prove those reactions, and help reveal the fact we are not all one-size-fits-all when it comes to hormones. For instance, why do some women gain weight on the pill, and others not at all? Our research will get us one step closer to discovering important and potentially novel biomarkers that may have an impact on individual responses to contraception.' They are looking for women or people assigned female at birth who have serious side effects, to try to work out why.

The sequencing will also be able to track and compare women of different ethnicities. For instance, South Asian women are more likely to get PCOS and Black women are more likely to get fibroids. 'Past contraceptive pill clinical trials were generally conducted on white women,' said

Elena, 'and other ethnicities might get entirely different side effects, better or worse, but no one has properly investigated that.' Dama is doing the first stage of genome mapping for free, with anonymised women who have donated their saliva and data, but eventually they will charge for the test, and they are hoping to bring the price down to a range similar to the ancestry tests.

Elena's co-founder is Paulina Cecula, a doctor at Imperial College NHS Trust in London. Dr Cecula's previous work included creating a chatbot that allows patients to ask essential medical questions before their contraception consultation, which has now been developed into a medical algorithm at Dama. Elena studied medical sciences and business at university, and I asked her if it had been hard to get investment for Dama. 'It's been a mix, but generally positive so far. We started our journey by pitching at Imperial for our first grant money, and the funding climate was a lot easier. Our first private investment round was successful, with investors reacting positively to our vision. When it comes to pitching the topic of contraception, I think male investors are a lot more aware of the problem than with other areas of women's health, because it affects them too, especially if they are in relationships – for example if their partner's sex drive has decreased from taking contraception.' She grinned.

THE HORMONAL DATA BANK

Dr Helen O'Neill, the CEO and founder of Hertility in London is also involved in the new FemTech movement.

She is a molecular geneticist and lecturer in women's health at University College London. She recognised that so many women worry about their hormone balance and whether or not they are fertile, particularly if their cycle has been masked by the pill for years. Hertility offers a simple blood test, which checks ten hormones including sex hormone binding globulin, testosterone, estrogen, and follicle stimulating hormone and they also take a detailed medical and symptom history, and as they build up data, identifying conditions like PCOS becomes clearer. 'We have about 140,000 blood samples so far, but it's in the amazing power of data and in interrogating data points as they cluster together that gives us the ability to predict different outcomes within the blood and the likelihood of having a condition.' When Hertility look at PCOS sufferers, and see that they don't ovulate, Dr O'Neill said they can suggest simple lifestyle changes which can sometimes help regain ovulation. They are also collaborating with the University of Edinburgh, looking at women with endometriosis.

Women can also see from the test whether there is a risk of premature ovarian insufficiency or early menopause. Dr O'Neill believes that the average age of menopause has become younger because we are exposed to endocrine disruptors. Obviously, it's a self-selecting group contacting Hertility, 'but we are seeing about a third of women under forty-five experiencing menopausal symptoms.' So many of the stories in this book began with women starting the pill in their early teens for acne or irregular periods.

'Often women just come off the pill and come to see us when they are thirty-five and have been on their pill for twenty years. They have never understood a regular cycle. Some of them don't even know whether they do have regular cycles. There is just a total silence around their bodies. And then they come off the pill hoping to kick-start these ovaries into action.'

Often women see that nothing is happening and go to a fertility clinic, 'but it's not in their best interest to find out what's wrong with you. It's in fertility clinics' best interest from a business perspective for them to sell you a package of three rounds of IVF.' (Hertility offers hormonal diagnoses, not IVF, although they do refer women to trusted doctors.) 'What's clear is that we need proper counselling for pre-conception care, and more so for anyone who is identifying as non-binary or trans, and taking gender-affirming hormones,' said Dr O'Neill. 'People need to know how their brains and bodies are working in this situation and understand what contraceptive hormones can do.'

BREAKING CONTRACEPTIVE NEWS

As well as better diagnoses, we need new contraceptives, as well as the male ones discussed in the previous chapter. Elizabeth Walden at MSI Reproductive Choices told me there has been talk for years about a once-a-month pill, taken either after a woman has had sex or has missed her period – closer to an abortion pill than the morning-after pill (which tends not to work after ovulation). The monthly pill would avoid women continuously having synthetic hormones in their bodies. But anti-abortion politics stand in the way of research.

Dr Lisa Haddad is the medical director of the Center for Biomedical Research at the Population Council in New York, and leads clinical development efforts on new methods. 'I know from my previous work at the bedside as an ObGyn that we need more choices for contraception to truly work. There are many diverse needs, and calls for non-hormonal methods for both men and women. We need to reduce side effects – which are the leading reason for discontinuation – for a better contraceptive experience, and if we can tackle HIV and STD [sexually transmitted disease] prevention at the same time, that would be perfect.'

The non-profit international Population Council works with pharmaceutical companies and is trialling a hormonal vaginal ring with the newer, low-side-effect progestin Nestorone, and another one with a progestin plus an anti-HIV compound. A pilot study is currently underway with twenty-four couples. There is also a non-hormonal, anti-STD vaginal ring in development that nukes HIV, chlamydia and gonorrhoea. This seems to be a top choice for the millions who ought to wear condoms on a one-night stand or early on in a relationship, but sometimes forget to do so. I didn't realise until I spoke to Dr Haddad that 63 per cent of new HIV infections are contracted by women and girls.[3]

She was also adamant, as a mother of two boys, that contraception should not solely be the responsibility of women, and there should be more research and development for men, including projects like Vasalgel (a temporary vasectomy) or the NES/T gel, a hormonal contraceptive for men. 'The untapped male contraception market is huge. We also need to prioritise and recognise unmet need in gender-diverse populations, and people with cognitive or physical disabilities. We need to dismantle assumptions around who uses contraception by consulting with diverse groups throughout the drug development process.'

Dr Haddad also thinks about the anthropology as well as the science. 'There could be products one day like fast-dissolving spermicidal inserts you could get in a vending machine in a bar. Then you don't have to negotiate with a partner or deal with the power dynamics of a condom.' The slow speed of development and regulation, is, however, frustrating. 'We need to treat contraception development with more urgency,' said Dr Haddad. 'My hope is to get to a place where women and men can control where and how they get pregnant, without negative effects.'

MALE ALLIES

Coming from the menopause space to the contraceptive space makes me *more* rather than less hopeful about male allyship and understanding. I give lots of talks to employees and management in factories, investment banks and the NHS about the menopause revolution, and I find the men who stand tentatively in suits at the back of the room relax and start to ask questions once they understand scientifically what the crash of hormones at menopause does to your brain, and how the majority of women can safely top up with body-identical HRT. They are empathetic and delighted that women can take action. Public enthusiasm for the male contraceptive gel and temporary vasectomy shows similar openness. I reckon if we knew more and spoke more about what hormonal contraception is doing to us, men would listen too, just as they have with the 'outing' of periods in the last decade or so. But that still means we're exposing ourselves, revealing our struggles as so many women have, on the record, in this book.

I was talking to my daughter Molly about this, and we agreed that perhaps men need to feel our pain. On the hormonal coil, she said, 'I still get excruciating cramps, but I have fewer, and they happen less often, and I don't know when they're coming. I do, however, find some solace in the TikTok channel that tests cramps on men, @getsomedays. That sounds really bad, but I'm thinking that my brothers have no idea. Sympathetic though they are, part of me would love for them to have a real physical understanding of what it means to have cramps. It's sort of like how you and I are exposing quite intimate parts of us here, and men don't have to. It's because I'm a woman. But it's also because I'm a woman that I feel the need to, because the healthcare world doesn't seem to get it. As Kristin Scott Thomas' character in the television series *Fleabag* says: 'women are born with pain built in . . . we carry it within ourselves our whole lives . . . men don't.' How do we still not understand ourselves? Or do we need every healthcare professional to have a cramp simulator put on them until they finally listen to us and do something about it?'

However, there are some men listening out there. One is friendly, bespectacled entrepreneur Frederik Petursson Madsen, CEO of Cirqle Biomedical in Denmark, who started researching better contraception for women after his girlfriend struggled. 'About eight years ago my girlfriend at the time told me that the pill was causing her mood swings. As a young guy, I didn't realise how common the side effects are. I quickly understood that I wouldn't want to use hormonal therapy myself, and was shocked by how limited the alternatives were and how little innovation there's been in contraception since the pill was introduced. So, coming from a business innovation background, I thought I'd try to find a solution. I talked with women to understand what an ideal contraceptive would look like, and then continued searching for a technology to create the best product.'

Fred started exploring the possibilities of creating a new kind of diaphragm that would be easier to use and more effective. Then he found Dr Thomas Crouzier, a scientist exploring ways to engineer mucus barriers. 'When we met, we realised that we could leverage the natural barrier that's already there, cervical mucus, and just strengthen it to prevent sperm penetration. In this way, we would simply mimic what happens outside of ovulation when the cervical mucus is thick and impenetrable for sperm.' They created a gel you put into the vagina before intercourse, which makes the natural mucus in the cervix impermeable to sperm and lasts for up to five hours afterwards.[4] The gel contains a natural biopolymer, which is used for blood clotting and wound healing, and when the gel is mixed with cervical mucus it thickens it — making sperm cells swim into a wall. Thickening mucus is also how the progestin pill works, so that makes sense.

The gel is different from spermicides, which have a high failure rate when used alone. Fred helpfully sent me a video of sperm in a petri dish crashing into the thickened mucus and bouncing back. 'The calm of a petri dish is rather different from the storm of sexual intercourse,' I said, but Fred explained that they tested the mucus barrier on thirty English and French ewes — plus some randy rams. 'None of the gel sheep got pregnant, but eight out of fifteen of the unprotected sheep conceived.' The successful initial research means the product now has a $10 million investment from Organon, a pharmaceutical company in women's health, who will do human trials if the research results are replicated at on a larger scale. Human trials will take three to five years.

WILL HORMONAL CONTRACEPTIVE RESEARCH MAKE A COMEBACK TOO?

While an on-demand, invisible, non-hormonal contraceptive will be a bedside holy grail for millions of women, there are others who still want to harness the positive and preventative effects of hormones in the pill, for heavy or no periods, acne, PCOS, endometriosis, PMS and PMDD. They also want better hormonal contraception, with a safer profile and fewer side effects. But research and approval are positively sluggardly around new methods of contraception, as Dr Haddad attested earlier. Why?

I asked Amanda Lee, the associate director of marketing at Theramex, a women's health pharmaceutical company, which also makes body-identical HRT and contraceptives. She has worked for twenty-five years in the industry in the UK, Australia and New Zealand. 'Years ago, I was working for Wyeth, who produced the HRT for the Women's Health Initiative, which then reported a link between [synthetic] HRT and breast cancer in 2002. It was a disaster.' Wyeth's stock plummeted by 24 per cent and millions were wiped off their shares. 'Basically research into hormones for women stopped, for the pill and HRT.

'There had been great research in the seventies and eighties, but everyone shelved it. There has been almost no research into new pills because the old ones are priced so low, you'd have to show amazing improvements to justify the extra cost – and how would you ever get your money back from millions spent on research?' Dr Haddad at the Population Council said she would like to see more women encouraged to go into medical research roles to reverse the male gaze in healthcare development, more government funding put towards treating conditions such as endometriosis, and better education in schools about what normal periods should be like. 'Things are already getting better,' she stresses. 'It's just we're reversing thousands of years of a patriarchal medical institution. It's like changing the direction of a cruise liner.'

FROM EXCLUSION TO INCLUSION

Think of every barrier we have discussed around contraception, and then build it even higher for racially and economically marginalised communities, trans and non-binary people, and people with disabilities. 'Disabilities' can mean a wide spectrum of functional, physical, sensory, or neurodivergent abilities that should not be allowed to stand in the way of sexual pleasure, self-determination, parenthood and accessible healthcare. A powerful article in the journal *Women's Health*[5] set out what needs sorting: 'We should engage in open-ended, shared decision-making about contraception and abortion, acknowledging that people with disabilities are the experts of their own health and bodies.' Clinics need to train staff on accessibility issues and equitable care, make sure there's better communication and more time, smash stereotypes, 'and address ableism in the field of medicine and their own practice, and assert that individuals with disabilities are whole, sexual beings'.

THE BODY-IDENTICAL HORMONE REVOLUTION

Everyone can benefit from the coming body-identical hormone revolution, pills which may be better tolerated and safer for women. Some changes are already afoot. Zoely came out in 2011, one of the new combined pills containing body-identical estrogens, and there is also Drovelis in 2021 from Mithra, and Qlaira in 2009 from Bayer. The three pills get higher ratings on The

Lowdown from users than the older combined pills like Rigevidon, but there are very small numbers of reviews so far, as they are not widely prescribed by the NHS but more available in Europe, America and Australia. Aside from the natural body-identical estrogen having a better effect on bone density, it also has a lower blood-clot risk than the synthetic ethinylestradiol in the usual combined pills,[6] as well as having a better effect on mental health, as explored in Chapter 3.[7]

Professor Jayashri Kulkarni of Monash University, Australia, has run trials on different progestins and depression,[8] especially on women with previous mood disorders, and said: 'Many of the older oral contraceptive pills, which contain ethinylestradiol, are linked to severe mood problems. Newer oral contraceptive pills containing natural estrogens can be better tolerated with a weaker link to mood problems. Doctors should be looking at this when they see someone's mood worsening on hormonal contraception.' There is also some research underway on whether the body-identical estrogens will be better tolerated by women who have monthly hormonal migraines when their estrogen dips after ovulation, and the new combined pill may help keep levels up with a lower risk of stroke or clot.[9]

Zoely and Qlaira contain E2, a copy of our natural estrogen, estradiol, but Drovelis contains E4, a copy of the estrogen estretrol, produced by the foetal liver, and it seems to work better at regulating unscheduled bleeding. Drovelis also contains the synthetic progestin drospirenone, found in Yasmin, which is good for acne prevention. Qlaira contains the progestin dienogest, and levels of hormones similar to the natural cycle, but with a two-day break, which helps women with heavy bleeding. Zoely's progestin, nomegestrol acetate, is longer-lasting in the body, so there is less of a risk when you miss a pill, and it tends not to lower libido.

So, there is a large menu of alternatives out there, but they are rarely offered as a first choice to women. The body-identical contraceptives are all approved by the NHS on the British National Formulary, but local areas may not list them, so you have to ask specially. As I was writing this, a friend who was having trouble with her pill went to ask for Drovelis instead, but her London GP had never heard of it, and it's not at the top of the prescribing list because it's more expensive. It's worth advocating for yourself and going in armed with research if your present pill doesn't suit you.

Because I use – and love – body-identical progesterone and estrogen in my HRT, I wondered why the safer progesterone (which has never been shown to increase the risk of breast cancer) is not used in contraception. Theramex already makes Zoely and a fully body-identical HRT pill called Bijuve, which contains estrogen and progesterone, which is also great for steadying women's hormones in perimenopause. Could they not make something similar for contraception? I got on the phone to Dr Mitra Boolell, head of medical affairs at Theramex. He explained that, so far, natural progesterone is not as reliable at inhibiting ovulation: 'Natural progesterone is not well absorbed compared to synthetic ones. But the micronized version, used in Bijuve, improves absorption. I think that natural progesterone will be there for contraception one day, but it will take time.' He sighed. 'If you want to save money on healthcare, don't save money on young women because they are the future of society.'

THE POSITIVE POWER OF HORMONES ON MENTAL HEALTH

We talk about 'tweakments' like Botox and fillers for our faces, but what about tweakments of our hormones to make our moods and lives better? Dr Katharina Dalton, the mother of research into premenstrual syndrome whom I mentioned earlier, used top-ups of progesterone to alleviate women's low mood in the later, luteal part of the cycle. At the University of Illinois at Chicago, clinical psychologist Dr Tory Eisenlohr-Moul works on groundbreaking research on cyclical mood disorders, and how titrating each individual's hormones can make a huge difference. 'I specialise in studying the effects of the menstrual cycle on emotions, thought patterns and behaviour in hormone-sensitive women, and I investigate how impulsive or dangerous behaviour such as suicide attempts, drug use, and verbal or physical conflict change across the cycle. My research is focused on identifying who's at risk for this hormone sensitivity, including trans and non-binary patients, and working out the hormonal and psychological variables that contribute to their symptoms.'

In one study, she tracked naturally-cycling psychiatric outpatients who had a history of suicidal thoughts in the past month. She provided natural estrogen patches and progesterone to one group in the two weeks before and during their period, and a placebo to a second group in the same time frame. (Eventually each participant was given a chance to try the placebo or the hormones.) The hormones (or placebo) were given around periods because that's during the time in the cycle when those hormones naturally drop.[10] Dr Eisenlohr-Moul questioned the participants about their moods in detailed surveys and asked them to track how they changed throughout their cycle. She concluded: 'We found that supplementing hormones in the two weeks before periods prevented premenstrual worsening of suicidal ideation, depressed mood, hopelessness, rejection sensitivity, perceived burdensomeness and perceived stress.'

But Dr Eisenlohr-Moul said that hormones were rarely taken into account by mainstream psychiatrists, and need to be flagged. 'It's really worth thinking about hormone supplementation for women with certain types of hormone sensitivity too. Some people have a major or small progesterone fluctuation sensitivity, some a small or large estrogen withdrawal sensitivity, some a bit of both.' I have one friend whose daughter uses a small pump of estrogen gel in the week leading up to her period, and that keeps migraines at bay, and we have also seen successful studies where a daily top-up of estrogen alleviates the crash of post-natal depression. Dr Eisenlohr-Moul concluded: 'I think part of the disservice that the medical community has done to women is that they haven't explored the complexity of different responses from each person.' We have new tools at our disposal in mental health, but they need to be taken out of the box.

LOOK AFTER YOUR DAUGHTERS

The thought that nagged me most often writing this book was around teenagers, and the cavalier way we put them on hormonal contraception not long after they learn to tie their shoelaces, at the stage when their bodies are growing and their minds are in the process of rewiring. Research has only just begun into how hormonal contraception affects brain formation, but we know it causes a more serious risk of depression in younger women, along with the other health risks. We need to look after our daughters. Dr O'Neill said: 'When your endocrine system is growing, it's this very dynamic orchestra of events happening through cross communication between your brain and ovaries, and what do we do? We cut off the connection between those parts at a time before the whole system has matured. It's quite staggering actually, to see the frequency with which we do that to teenagers.'

Of course, a girl with tsunami periods deserves medical help, and we need the safest possible contraception for those who cannot find their homework, never mind their pills, but is there a better way for some? Irregular periods are perfectly normal at first, and for many, they don't settle down for a few years. Also, the blanket use of synthetic hormones to prevent acne is sometimes unnecessary – there are other options. Teaching young teenagers to use an app like Clue to track their cycle, get comfortable with it, and anticipate mood swings and periods would be a very good use of school science classes – for girls, and boys observing, and non-binary kids – as would explaining to young scientists what ingredients are in the hormonal contraception they are about to use. It's far more use than dissecting a frog. Presently, sex education is shocking in its impracticality. So be with your daughters, your sisters, or your friends on the hormonal contraception journey, and make sure they get the best help — and not the bog-standard version. A Flo app survey showed women aged eighteen to twenty-four were nearly ten times more likely than women aged forty-four to fifty-five to turn to social media for reproductive health information, so make sure the teenagers in your life are armed with scientific truth and not wild rumour.

MOVE FAST AND BREAK THINGS

Melinda Gates, who was once married to one of those 'move fast and break things' tech bros, now uses her fortune to advance women's health and said: 'Contraceptives are the greatest life-saving, poverty-ending, women-empowering innovation ever created.' She pointed out that there are still 214 million women and girls in developing countries who cannot get access to the contraceptives they want. 'In fact, no country in the last fifty years has emerged from poverty without expanding access to contraceptives.'[11]

So we still need to move fast and break things for there to be a real pillquake across the world. The contraception business was patriarchal and sclerotic, so we must make it more innovative and erotic. Since the days when the pill was first tested on women in an insane asylum and in the slums of Puerto Rico, the history of contraception has been of one long medical experiment on women, who often had no idea what they were putting into their bodies. At last we know precisely what hormonal contraception contains, and how it possesses our bodies and brains. It's time to reclaim contraception's powers for our own good, and our own health. Now that you've read *Everything You Need to Know About The Pill*, please don't leave it sitting on a dusty bookshelf. Pass it on to a friend, a colleague, or a daughter. Or leave it on a park bench for a stranger. Start a conversation that we should have had half a century ago.

ACKNOWLEDGEMENTS

So many people have given so much time to help connect humanity and science in this book: doctors, academics and experts, and above all the women who have told their stories with hindsight, insight and devastating honesty. Thank you for letting me listen.

My biggest thanks goes to the catalyst for this investigation: my daughter Molly Macintyre, who not only told her own story but opened my eyes to what was happening to a whole generation out there, and helped kick-start the research.

The backbone of this work comes from dozens of doctors and healthcare professionals – both those who advised on background and those who are quoted – who all generously shared their years of expertise. Thanks to Dr Gail Allsopp, Dr Julia Bailey, Dr Janet Barter, Dr Mitra Boolell, Dr Lynae Brayboy, Dr Sally Darnborough, Dr Tory Eisenlohr-Moul, Rebecca Elderfield, Katharine Gale, Dr Lisa Haddad, Dr Therese Johansson, Dr Jayne Kavanagh, Prof Jayashri Kulkarni, Dr Søren Vinther Larsen, Professor Øjvind Lidegaard, Dr Diana Mansour,

Dr Yvonne Neubauer, Dr Helen O'Neill, Professor Dame Lesley Regan, Dr Dan Reisel, Simphiwe Sesane, Dr Charlotte Skovlund, Dr Carys Sonneberg, Dr Annabel Sowemimo, Professor Judith Stevenson, Mr Vikram Sinai Talaulikar and last but not least, Dr Louise Newson, who over the last few years has shown me medicine through a new and radical lens.

Then there are the storytellers: the women, men, non-binary and trans people who spoke so movingly of their experiences. Huge thanks to: Suzie Bishop, Lauren Chiren, Tessa Clemson, Jody Coyle, Eloise Donovan, Abby Fry, Dan and Emily Glastonbury, Kirsty Keating, Asha Knight, Holly McComish, Jennifer Moore, Maya Oppenheim, Laura Price, Christine Purkis, Anna Robertson, Aisha Torabally, Kate Walsh, Dee Whitnell, Hannah Wrathall – and all the Instagrammers.

So many experts, campaigners and academics also contributed and advised, particularly the staff of Brook and MSI Reproductive Choices, as well as Professor Richard Anderson, Tina Backhouse, Elena Rueda Carrasco, Jean-Manuel Fontaine, R.L. Fox, Neelam Heera-Shergill, Dr Sarah E. Hill, Amanda Lee, Frederik Madsen, Priya Lakhani-Quiling, Sarah Panzetta, Alice Pelton, Natasha Richardson, Professor Craig Roberts, Jennifer Takhar, and Dr Caitlin Taylor.

My conversation with Molly led to us pitching a pill documentary to Channel 4. With the expert guidance of executive producer Katie Lander at Finestripe Productions in Glasgow, that proposal became *Davina McCall's Pill Revolution* in 2023. Thanks to Joanna Potts and Leah

Green at Channel 4, to Davina for always being a trooper and a revolutionary, and to director Alice McShane and assistant producer Charlotte Hall for all their hard work and research.

Thanks to my wonderful agent, Sheila Crowley at Curtis Brown, for steering and encouraging all these women's health projects; to my commissioning editor at Simon & Schuster, Alison MacDonald, and my editors Sophia Akhtar and Kat Ailes for cheerfully bearing with a baggy, complicated manuscript; to the marketing and publicity team Harriett Collins, Laurie McShea, Sabah Khan and Hannah Paget; to Jenny Smith for my author photograph; and to my publisher, Suzanne Baboneau.

On the home front, thanks to James Scott, for the science and to Katie Scott for her help with research. Once again, I'm grateful to my sons Finn and Barney Macintyre for suggestions, support and general entertainment, and to Cameron Scott, my partner, for his love, tolerance, and ability to keep me relatively sane.

FURTHER RESOURCES

@pillscandal
Regular updates on contraception, gender bias, and the latest science from Kate Muir on Instagram, Twitter/X and TikTok.

Brook
Brook is a charity supporting people with their sexual health, contraception and well-being, with a user-friendly website and clinics.
www.brook.org.uk

Contraception Choices
University College London site with honest information on the pros and cons of different contraceptives.
www.contraceptionchoices.org

Faculty of Sexual and Reproductive Healthcare
Up-to-date detailed information on contraception and sexual health for professionals, but also useful for the general reader.
www.fsrh.org.uk

The Lowdown
The 'Trip Advisor' for contraception with user reviews and advice from doctors. Also sells many brands of pill.
www.thelowdown.com

MSI Reproductive Choices

An international organisation providing safe abortions and contraception. NHS-funded and private abortion and vasectomy care through a network of local clinics across England.
www.msichoices.org.uk

National Health Service

NHS information and advice on contraception, abortion and sexual health.
www.nhs.uk/conditions/contraception/
www.nhs.uk/conditions/abortion/

Planned Parenthood USA

Contraception, abortion, pregnancy and sexual health care and advice across America.
www.plannedparenthood.org

National Abortion Hotline USA

Toll-free, multilingual hotline for abortion provider information and financial assistance in the US and Canada (1-800-772-9100).
www.prochoice.org

Sexwise

Honest advice about contraception, pregnancy, sexually transmitted infections and pleasure.
www.sexwise.org.uk

Reproductive Justice Initiative

Formerly Decolonising Contraception, this is a charity with a radical approach to reproductive health and rights which that seeks to address complex social, economic and political factors.
www.reprojusticeinitiative.org

Cysters

A collective changing the narrative around reproductive and mental well-being, striving for equal access to healthcare for

marginalized communities and people of colour.
www.cysters.org

Dean St

Website and London clinic focusing on the needs of the LGBTQI+ community, offering contraceptive and sexual health care.
www.dean.st

CliniQ

Offers a holistic sexual health, mental health and well-being service for trans, non-binary and gender-diverse people.
www.cliniq.org

Wellbeing of Women

Charity researching, educating and campaigning on women's health, which also runs events.
www.wellbeingofwomen.org.uk

Endometriosis UK

Charity supporting people with endometriosis.
www.endometriosis-uk.org

Verity-PCOS UK

Charity supporting people with polycystic ovarian syndrome.
www.verity-pcos.org.uk

International Association for Premenstrual Disorders

Provides support, information and resources for anyone impacted by premenstrual disorders like PMDD.
www.iapmd.org

NOTES

CHAPTER 1

1 'Contraception Poll' for *Pill Revolution* on Channel 4, https://savanta.com, June 2023.
2 *Fleabag*, Episode 2, https://www.youtube.com/watch?v=mRuSDZkhO-M, 2019.
3 'Contraception Poll', https://savanta.com, June 2023.
4 United Nations, 'Contraceptive Use by Method 2019 Data Booklet', January 2019.
5 'Abortion statistics, England and Wales: 2021', gov.uk, October 2023; 'Termination of pregnancy statistics', https://public
   healthscotland.scot, May 2023.
6 Schoenfeld Walker, A. and McCann, A., 'Abortions rose in most states this year, new data shows', https://www.nytimes.com, September 2023.
7 Tiktoks in *Disclosure: Should I Quit My Birth Control*, https://www.bbc.co.uk, September 2023.
8 NewsGuard Misinformation Monitor: September 2022, 'Beware the "New Google": TikTok's search engine pumps toxic misinformation to its young users', https://www.newsguardtech.com/misinformation-monitor/september-2022/
9 Schneider-Kamp, A., Takhar, J., 'Interrogating the pill: Rising distrust and the reshaping of health risk perceptions

in the social media age', *Social Science & Medicine*, Vol 331, August 2023.

10   https://www.nhs.uk/conditions/contraception/
     combined-contraceptive-pill/

11   Martin, D., Timmons, K. et al, 'Injury Incidence Across
     the Menstrual Cycle in International Footballers', *Frontiers in
     Sports and Active Living*, 616999, August 18, 2021.

12   'Contraception Poll', https://savanta.com, June 2023.

13   'Oestrogen and progestogen effects of COC', https://
     gpnotebook.com, March 2021.

14   https://thelowdown.com

15   'FSRH Clinical Guideline: Contraceptive Choices for
     Young People', https://www.fsrh.org/documents/cec-ceu-
     guidance-young-people-mar-2010/, amended, May 2019.

16   'Breaking point: Securing the future of sexual health
     services', https://www.local.gov.uk, November 2022.

17   FOIs for *Pill Revolution* programme, June 2023.

18   https://assets.publishing.service.gov.uk/media/
     60ed6a7bd3bf7f56801f3ca1/ROI_LARC_maternity.pdf

19   https://www.kff.org/womens-health-policy/fact-sheet/
     womens-health-insurance-coverage/, December 2022.

20   'Contraception Poll', https://savanta.com, June 2023.

21   Tapper, J., 'Revealed: huge disparities in birth control
     prescriptions across England', https://www.theguardian.
     com, June 2023.

22   Heera-Shergill, N., 'Let's change the narrative made for us
     and reclaim our own identity', https://www.youtube.com/
     watch?v=jyOAIgkid9w, 2019.

23   Janjua, H., 'Taliban fighters stop chemists selling
     contraception', https://www.theguardian.com, February
     2023.

CHAPTER 2

1   Gross, R., 'Why Women on the Pill Still "Need" to Have
    Their Periods', https://www.nytimes.com, December 2019.

2 'Contraception Poll', https://savanta.com, June 2023.

3 Percy, L., Mansour, D., *Contraception Made Easy*, (Banbury, Scion, 2015)

4 Gorman, T., *No, Prime Minister!*, (Kingston upon Thames, John Blake, 2011), p. 275.

5 https://www.nhs.uk/conditions/contraception/
the-pill-progestogen-only/

6 'Contraception Poll', https://savanta.com, June 2023.

7 https://www.contraceptionchoices.org

8 Guillebaud, J., MacGregor, A., 'The 7-day contraceptive hormone-free interval should be consigned to history', *BMJ Sexual & Reproductive Health*, 2017, 200036.

9 Guillebaud, J., MacGregor, A., *Contraception: Your Questions Answered 7ed*, (Oxford, Elsevier, 2017)

10 Parkhill, T., 'Mood dips during pill pause', https://www.neurosciencenews.com, September 2023.

11 MacGregor, A., 'The Pill: Consigning the 7-day pill-free interval to history', https://www.annemacgregor.com, July 2018.

12 https://womenshistory.si.edu/herstory/health-wellness/
object/ortho-dialpak-oral-contraceptive

13 https://americanhistory.si.edu/explore/stories/
50th-anniversary-pill

14 http://www.fawcettsociety.org.uk/news/landmark-study-menopausal-women-let-down-by-employers-and-healthcare-providers May 2022.

15 https://www.wellbeingofwomen.org.uk/what-we-do/
campaigns/just-a-period/

16 'Contraception Poll', https://savanta.com, June 2023.

17 Maisie Hill, *Period Power*, (London, Green Tree, 2019).

18 Panay N., Fenton A., 'The role of testosterone in women', *Climacteric*, 2009, 12, 185–187.

19 https://www.nhs.uk/conditions/pre-menstrual-syndrome/

20 'Body identical hormones', https://www.balance-menopause.com, August 2023. https://www.balance-menopause.com/menopause-library/
body-identical-hormones-factsheet/#:~:text=Body-

identical-progesterone-treatments&text=This-has-fewer-side,Mirena-coil-receive-progestogen.

21 Giatti, S., Melcangi, R., Pesaresi, M., 'The other side of progestins: effects in the brain', *Journal of Molecular Endocrinology*, 57 (2), 109–126.

22 Clue App, https://www.helloclue.com.

23 Faculty of Sexual and Reproductive Healthcare website, https://www.fsrh.org.

24 Larsen, S., Köhler-Forsberg, K., et al, 'Oral contraceptives and the serotonin 4 receptor: a molecular brain imaging study in healthy women', *Acta Psychiatrica Scandinavica*, 2020, 142(4), 294–306.

25 Lovett, J., Chima, M., et al, 'Oral contraceptives cause evolutionarily novel increases in hormone exposure', *Evolution, Medicine, and Public Health*, 2017(1), 97–108.

26 https://www.niddk.nih.gov/health-information/health-statistics/overweight-obesity

27 https://www.plannedparenthood.org/blog/does-the-pill-make-you-gain-weight

28 https://www.nhs.uk/conditions/contraception/combined-contraceptive-pill/

29 Lopez, L., Ramesh, S., et al, 'Progestin-only contraceptives: effects on weight, *Cochrane Database of Systematic Reviews*, 2016(8), CD008815.

30 Gallo, M., Lopez L., et al, 'Combination contraceptives: effects on weight', *Cochrane Database of Systematic Reviews, v* 2014 (1), CD003987.

31 https://www.nhs.uk/medicines/contraceptive-injections-medroxyprogesterone/common-questions-about-medroxyprogesterone-contraceptive-injections/

32 Patient Leaflet, Microgynon 30, https://www. medicines. org, February 2023.

33 'Progestin-Only Hormonal Birth Control: Pill and Injection', https://www.acog.org/womens-health/faqs/progestin-only-hormonal-birth-control-pill-and-injection, January 2023.

34 Jaffe, L., 'Is Bone Health at Risk for Adolescents on Birth Control?', https://www.medcentral.com/endocrinology/osteoporosis/bone-health-risk-adolescents-birth-control, September 2020.

CHAPTER 3

1 'Davina McCall calls for revolution on contraception', https://www.independent.co.uk, June 2023.
2 'Birth Control Pill', https://www.plannedparenthood.org/learn/birth-control/birth-control-pill.
3 https://www.nhs.uk/conditions/contraception/combined-contraceptive-pill/
4 Patient Leaflet for Dianette, https://www.medicines.org.uk, February 2023.
5 ibid.
6 Lovett, J., Chima, M., et al. 'Oral contraceptives cause evolutionarily novel increases in hormone exposure: A risk factor for breast cancer', *Evolution, Medicine, and Public Health*, 2017, 97–108.
7 Faculty of Sexual and Reproductive Healthcare website, https://www.fsrh.org.
8 'FSRH Clinical Guideline: Progestogen-only Pills (August 2022, Amended July 2023', https://www.fsrh.org/documents/cec-guideline-pop/
9 'Mood change is common and often related to external events', https://www.fsrh.org, July 2023.
10 https://thl.fi/en/web/thlfi-en/-/the-number-of-abortions-is-decreasing-in-the-nordic-countries-finland-s-abortion-rate-still-lowest, March 2023.
11 Skovlund, C., Mørch, L., Kessing, L., Lidegaard, Ø, 'Association of Hormonal Contraception with Depression', *JAMA Psychiatry*, 2016, 73(11), 1154–1162.
12 "Not shown the contraception–depression link," https://www.fsrh.org, July 2023.
13 Skovlund, C., Mørch, L., et al. 'Association of Hormonal

Contraception With Suicide Attempts and Suicides', *The American Journal of Psychiatry*, 2018, 175(4), 336–342.

14 'Depression risk in users of different doses of levonorgestrel intrauterine systems: a nationwide prospective cohort study', Skovlund, C. W. et al., The Lancet Regional Health – Europe, thelancet.com, January 2024, 100813.

15 Patient Leaflet for Cerazette 75, https://www.medicines.org. uk, April 2022.

16 'Whether the hormonal contraception is the cause of these changes', https://www.fsrh.org, May 2019.

17 Johansson, T., Larsen, S., et al, 'Select Population-based cohort study of oral contraceptive use and risk of depression', *Epidemiology and Psychiatric Sciences*, 2023, 32, published online by Cambridge University Press.

18 Costa-Ramón, A., Daysal, M., et al, 'The Oral Contraceptive Pill and Adolescents' Mental Health', 2023, https://www.ssrn.com, IZA discussion paper 16288.

19 Lundin, C., Wikman, A., et al, 'There is no association between combined oral hormonal contraceptives and depression: a Swedish register-based cohort study', *British Journal of Obstetrics and Gynaecology*, 2022, 129(6), 917–925.

20 Zethraeus N., Dreber A., Ranehill E., et al, 'A first-choice combined oral contraceptive influences general well-being in healthy women: a double-blind, randomized, placebo-controlled trial, *Fertility and Sterility,* 2017, 107, 1238–45.

21 De Wit, A., De Vries, Y., et al, 'Hormonal contraceptive use and depressive symptoms: systematic review and network meta-analysis of randomised trials', *BJ Psych Open,* 2021, 7(4), e110.

22 Santer, M., Lawrence M., et al, 'Effectiveness of spironolactone for women with acne vulgaris (SAFA) in England and Wales',*BMJ,* 2023 *381, e074349.*

23 https://www.fda.gov/drugs/drug-safety-and-availability/ fda-drug-safety-communication-updated-information-about-risk-blood-clots-women-taking-birth-control

24 'Bayer's Yasmin Lawsuit Settlements Rise to $402.6 Million', bloomberg.com, July 2012.

25 'Yaz / Yasmin Drug Side Effects Class Action', https://www.clg.org.

26 Grigg-Spall, H., *Sweetening The Pill: Or how we got hooked on hormonal birth control*, (London, Zero Books, 2013).

27 ibid 6—7.

28 ibid 9.

29 https://www.podcasts.apple.com/ie/podcast/dwc-049-the-business-of-birth-control-with-holly/id1267527313?i=1000579161511

30 *The Business of Birth Control* film, https://www.thebusinessof.life, 2023.

31 https://www.sweeteningthepill.com/workshops/632-2/

32 Mu E., Kulkarni J., 'Hormonal contraception and mood disorders', *Australian Prescriber*, 2022, 45(3), 75—79.

33 Larsen, S., Köhler-Forsberg, K., 'Oral contraceptives and the serotonin 4 receptor: a molecular brain imaging study in healthy women', *Acta Psychiatrica Scandinavica*, 142 (4), 294—306.

34 Mu E., Kulkarni J., 'Hormonal contraception and mood disorders', *Australian Prescriber*, 2022, 45(3), 75—79.

CHAPTER 4

1 https://flo.health/landings/reproductive-health-report-uk, May, 2023.

2 Guillebaud, J., *Contraception Your Questions Answered* (5th Ed) (London, Churchill Livingstone, 2008).

3 Percy, L., Mansour, D., *Contraception Made Easy*, (Banbury, Scion, 2015).

4 ibid 67 and 77.

5 ibid 52.

6 Pastor Z., Holla K., Chmel R., 'The influence of combined oral contraceptives on female sexual desire: a systematic review'. *European Journal of Contraception and Reproductive Health Care*, 2013,18(1), 27—43.

7 Zethraeus N., Dreber, A., et al. 'Combined Oral

Contraceptives and Sexual Function in Women – a Double-Blind, Randomized, Placebo-Controlled Trial', *The Journal of Clinical Endocrinology and Metabolism*, 2016, 101(11), 4046–4053.

8   Raudrant D., Rabe T., 'Progestogens with antiandrogenic properties', *Drugs* 2003, 63, 463–492.

9   Skrzypulec V., Drosdzol A., 'Evaluation of quality of life and sexual functioning of women using levonorgestrel-releasing intrauterine contraceptive system Mirena', *Collegium Antropologicum*, 2008, 32(4), 1059–1068.

10 De Castro Coelho F., Barros C., 'The Potential of Hormonal Contraception to Influence Female Sexuality', *International Journal of Reproductive Medicine*, 2019, 9701384.

11 Boozalis A., Tutlam N., et al, 'Sexual Desire and Hormonal Contraception' *Obstetrics & Gynecology*, 2016, 127(3), 563–572.

12 McCarthy, M., 'I have the jab so I can't be blamed for getting pregnant', *Women's Studies International Forum*, 2009, 32930, 198–208.

13 'Depo-Provera and bone health', https://theros.org.uk, April 2017.

14 Vinogradova, Y., Coupland, C., 'Use of hormone replacement therapy and risk of breast cancer: nested case-control studies using the QResearch and CPRD databases', *BMJ*, 2020, 371, m3873.

15 McFarland, L., 'Depo-Provera Therapy as an Alternative to Imprisonment', *Houston Law Review*, 1986, 23(3) 801–819.

16 Panzer, C., Wise, S., et al, 'Women's Sexual Dysfunction: Impact of Oral Contraceptives on Sex Hormone-Binding Globulin and Androgen Levels', *Journal of Sexual Medicine*, 2006, 3(1) 104–113.

17 Panzer, C., 'The use of oral contraceptives . . .', https://www. sciencedaily.com, January 2006.

18 Bakus, C., Budge, K., et al. 'The impact of contraceptives on the vaginal microbiome in the non-pregnant state', *Frontiers in Microbiomes*, 2023, 1 1055472.

19   Spinillo A., Capuzzo E., et al, 'The impact of oral
      contraception on vulvovaginal candidiasis', *Contraception*,
      1995, 51(5), 293–7.

20   Handy, A., McMahon L., et al, 'Reduction in genital sexual
      arousal varies by type of oral contraceptive pill', *The Journal
      of Sexual Medicine*, 2023, 20(8), 094–1102.

21   https://thelowdown.com.

22   https://www.nhs.uk/conditions/vulvodynia/

23   Aerts L., Pluchino N., 'Hormonal contraception and
      vulvodynia: an update', *Gynecological and Reproductive
      Endocrinology & Metabolism,* 2021, 03, 156–161.

24   Labrie F., Archer D., et al, 'Efficacy of intravaginal
      dehydroepiandrosterone (DHEA) on moderate to severe
      dyspareunia and vaginal dryness, symptoms of vulvovaginal
      atrophy, and of the genitourinary syndrome of menopause',
      Menopause, 2016, 23(3), 243–56.

25   London, A., Klipping C., et al, 'Estetrol Combined with
      Drospirenone: An Investigational Oral Contraceptive With
      A Selective Impact on Endocrine Parameters', *The Journal of
      Sexual Medicine*, 20 (30), qdad068.013.

26   Caruso, S., Agnello, C., et al, 'Preliminary study on the
      effect of four-phasic estradiol valerate and dienogest (E2V/
      DNG) oral contraceptive on the quality of sexual life', *The
      Journal of Sexual Medicine*, 2011, 8(10), 2841–50.

27   Burke A., 'Nomegestrol acetate-17b-estradiol for oral
      contraception', *Patient Preference and Adherence*, 2013, 7,
      607–19.

28   Newson, L., Scott, A., 'Should we be prescribing
      testosterone to perimenopausal and menopausal women?
      A guide to prescribing testosterone for women in primary
      care', *British Journal of General Practice*, 2020, 70 (693),
      203–204.

29   https://freudpage.info.

CHAPTER 5

1   Roberts, C., Gosling, M., et al, 'MHC-correlated odour preferences in humans and the use of oral contraceptives,' *Proceedings of the Royal Society B*, 2008, 2715–2722.

2   Little, A., Burriss, R., et al, 'Oral contraceptive use in women changes preferences for male facial masculinity and is associated with partner facial masculinity', *Psychoneuroendocrinology,* 2013, 38(9),1777–85.

3   Miller, G., Tybur, J., Jordan, B., 'Ovulatory cycle effects on tip earnings by lap dancers: economic evidence for human estrus?', *Evolution and Human Behavior,* 2007, 28, 375–381.

4   Miller, S., Maner, J., 'Scent of a Woman: Men's Testosterone Responses to Olfactory Ovulation Cues', *Psychological Science,* 21(2), 276–283.

5   Strom, J., Ingberg, E., et al, 'The female menstrual cycle does not influence testosterone concentrations in male partners', *Journal of Negative Results in Biomedicine,* 2012, 11:1.

6   Tarumi, W., Shinohara, K., 'Women's body odour during the ovulatory phase modulates testosterone and cortisol levels in men', *PLoS One,* 2020, 15(3), e0230838.

7   Batres, C., Porcheron, A., et al, 'Evidence That the Hormonal Contraceptive Pill Is Associated With Cosmetic Habits' *Frontiers in Psychology*, 2018, 9, 1459.

8   https://www.thepinknews.com/2023/01/09/woman-contraceptive-pill-gay-tessa-bo/, January 2023.

9   Roberts, C., Klapilová, K. et al., 'Relationship satisfaction and outcome in women who meet their partner while using oral contraception', *Proceedings of the Royal Society B*, 2012, 279(1732), 1430–6.

10   Gangestad, S., Thornhill, R., 'Menstrual cycle variation in women's preferences for the scent of symmetrical men', *Proceedings of the Royal Society B*, 1998, 265(1399), 927–33.

11   Garza, R., Byrd-Craven, J., 'The role of hormones in attraction and visual attention to facial masculinity', *Frontiers in Psychology*, 2023, Sec. Evolutionary Psychology, 14.

12 Hill, S., *How the Pill Changes Everything: Your brain on birth control*, (London, Orion Spring, 2019), 119.

13 ibid, 89.

14 Follesa, P., Porcu, P., et al, 'Changes in GABAA receptor gamma 2 subunit gene expression induced by long-term administration of oral contraceptives in rats', *Neuropharmacology*, 2002, 42(3), 325–36.

15 Petersen, N., Beltz, A. M., Casto, K.V., et al, 'Towards a more comprehensive neuroscience of hormonal contraceptives', *Nature Neuroscience*, 2023, 26, 529–531.

16 Pletzer, B., 'Sex Hormones and Gender Role Relate to Gray Matter Volumes in Sexually Dimorphic Brain Areas', *Frontiers in Neuroscience*, 2019, 13, 592.

17 Pletzer, B., Kronbichler, M., Kerschbaum, H., 'Differential effects of androgenic and anti-androgenic progestins on fusiform and frontal gray matter volume and face recognition performance', *Brain Research*, 2015, 1596, 108–15.

18 Menting-Henry, S., Hildago-Lopez, E., 'Oral Contraceptives Modulate the Relationship Between Resting Brain Activity, Amygdala Connectivity and Emotion Recognition – A Resting State fMRI Study' *Frontiers in Behavioral Neuroscience*, 2022, Sec. Behavioral Endocrinology, 16.

19 Koebele, S., Poisson, M., 'Evaluating the Cognitive Impacts of Drospirenone, a Spironolactone-Derived Progestin, Independently and in Combination With Ethinyl Estradiol in Ovariectomized Adult Rats', *Frontiers in Neuroscience*, 2022, Sec. Neuroendocrine Science, 16.

20 https://scitechdaily.com/scientists-discover-new-side-effect-of-birth-control-pills/, August 2023.

21 Giatti, S., Melcangi, R., Pesare, M., 'The other side of progestins: effects in the brain', *Journal of Molecular Endodrinology*, 2016, 57(2), 109–126.

CHAPTER 6

1   https://time.com/6200542/women-birth-control-switching-methods-abortion/, July 2022.

2   https://www.britannica.com/science/Dalkon-Shield

3   thelowdown.com/all-reviews

4   https://helloclue.com/articles/sex/how-do-iuds-prevent-pregnancy, October 2019.

5   Costescu, D., Chawla, R., Hughes, R., et al, 'Discontinuation rates of intrauterine contraception due to unfavourable bleeding: a systematic review', *BMC Women's Health,* 2022, 22, 82.

6   Akintomide, H., Barnes, P., et al, 'Higher discontinuation rate with a standard-sized compared to a small-sized "gold standard" copper intrauterine device: a case-control review', *BMJ Sexual & Reproductive Health*, 2019, 200296. doi: 10.1136/bmjsrh-2018-200296.

7   Curtis, K., Jatlaoui, T., Tepper, N., et al, 'U.S. Selected Practice Recommendations for Contraceptive Use', *MMWR Recommendations and Reports,* 2016, 65(RR-4), 1–66.

8   Mørch, L., Skovlund, C., 'Contemporary Hormonal Contraception and the Risk of Breast Cancer', *The New England Journal of Medicine,* 2017, 377, 2228–2239.

9   'Mayo Clinic Q and A: Risk factors for uterine fibroids', https://newsnetwork.mayoclinic.org, October 2018.

10 'Landmark study: menopausal women let down by employers and healthcare providers', https://www.fawcettsociety.org.uk, May 2022.

11 https://www.accessdata.fda.gov, August 2022.

12 'Rosenberg, M., Meyers, A., Roy, V., 'Efficacy, cycle control, and side effects of low- and lower-dose oral contraceptives', *Contraception,* 1999, 60, (6), 321–329.

13 Hubacher, D., Chen, P., Park, S., 'Side effects from the copper IUD: do they decrease over time?' *Contraception,* 2009, 79(5), 356–62.

14 https://www.accessdata.accessdata.fda.gov, August 2020.

15 Mu, E., Kulkarni, J., 'Hormonal contraception and mood disorders', *Australian Prescriber*, 2022, 45(3), 75–79.

16 Zeiss, R., Schönfeldt-Lecuona, C., et al, 'Depressive Disorder With Panic Attacks After Replacement of an Intrauterine Device Containing Levonorgestrel: A Case Report', *Frontiers in Psychiatry*, 2020,11:561685.

17 Totten, M., Davenport, T., et al, 'Trace Minerals and Anxiety: A Review of Zinc, Copper, Iron, and Selenium' *Dietetics*, 2023, 2(1), 83–103.

18 Slattery, J., Morales, D., et al, 'Cohort Study of Psychiatric Adverse Events Following Exposure to Levonorgestrel-Containing Intrauterine Devices in UK General Practice', *Drug Safety*, 2018, 41(10), 951–958.

19 https://www.thetimes.co.uk/article/i-thought-my-coil-was-making-me-mad-3jnl9qs56, May 2023.

20 Buhling, K., Zite, N., et al, 'Worldwide use of intrauterine contraception: a review' *Contraception*, 2014, 89 (3), 162–173.

21 https://www.theguardian.com/society/2021/sep/24/viral-tiktok-video-of-iud-removal-at-home-prompts-warning-from-health-authorities, September 2021.

22 @d_m_r82

23 @Femalehealthdoc

24 @Thesocialmenopause

25 'Vasovagal syncope', mayoclinic.org, March 2023.

26 https://www.nhs.uk/conditions/contraception/iud-coil/

27 'The Endometriosis Society says coils have been shown to help with period pain', endometriosis.org, April 2011.

28 https://www.fsrh.org, March 2023.

29 Hall, A., Kutler, B., 'Intrauterine contraception in nulliparous women: a prospective survey', *Journal of Family Planning and Reproductive Health Care*, 2016, 42(1), 36–42.

30 https://cdphe.colorado.gov/fpp/about-us/colorados-success-long-acting-reversible-contraception-larc, January 2017.

31 Buhling, K., Zite, N., et al, 'Worldwide use of intrauterine contraception: a review' *Contraception*, 2014, 89 (3), 162–173.

32 https://www.plannedparenthood.org/learn/birth-control/iud/how-can-i-get-an-iud

CHAPTER 7

1 Mantel, H., 'Every part of my body hurt', June 2004, https://www.theguardian.com/society/2004/jun/07/health.genderissues

2 Dunham, L., 'In Her Own Words: Lena Dunham on Her Decision to Have a Hysterectomy at 31', https://www.vogue.com/article/lena-dunham-hysterectomy-vogue-march-2018-issue, March 2018.

3 https://www.wrh.ox.ac.uk/news/endometriosis-black-women-continue-to-receive-poorer-care-for-the-condition, March 2023.

4 Monnin, N., Fattet, A., Koscinski, I., 'Endometriosis: Update of Pathophysiology, (Epi) Genetic and Environmental Involvement' *Biomedicines*, 2023, 11(3), 978.

5 Vercellini, P., Buggio, L., Berlanda, N., et al. 'Estrogen-progestins and progestins for the management of endometriosis', *Fertility and Sterility*, 2016,106,1552–1571.

6 Muzii, L., Di Tucci, C., et al, 'Continuous versus cyclic oral contraceptives after laparoscopic excision of ovarian endometriomas: a systematic review and meta-analysis', *American Journal of Obstetrics and Gynecology*, 2016, 214(2), 203–211.

7 https://www.theguardian.com/society/2023/oct/18/naga-munchetty-i-was-failed-and-gaslit-by-nhs-despite-debilitating-periods-and-symptoms, October 2023.

8 https://www.theguardian.com/society/2023/may/22/naga-munchetty-pain-womb-condition-adenomyosis, May 2023.

9 https://www.fsrh.org, September 2019.

10 'Women's Troubles', https://harpers.org, April 2018.

11 'Global study shows the experience of Endometriosis is rooted in genetics', https://www.ox.ac.uk, March 2023.

12 MacDonald, A., 'Diagnosing Endometriosis Using Menstrual Blood', Technology Networks, March 2020.

13   https://www.larabriden.com/guide-to-using-progesterone-
     for-womens-health/, February 2023.

14   https://www.larabriden.com/endometriosis-treat-the-
     immune-system/, February 2022.

15   'Researchers optimistic about potential new treatment for
     endometriosis.', Guardian.com, March 2023.

16   Martín-Merino, E., Wallander, M., et al, 'The reporting
     and diagnosis of uterine fibroids in the UK: an observational
     study' *BMC Womens Health*, 2016, 25 (16) 45.

17   https://www.contemporaryobgyn.net, May 2023.

18   https://bwhi.org/2019/04/03/its-not-normal-black-women-
     stop-suffering-from-fibroids/, April 2019.

19   'I've been on the waitlist for over a year: Britain is in the grip
     of a gynaecological crisis', https://www.independent.co.uk/
     life-style/health-and-families/gynaecologist-uk-waiting-
     times-nhs-b2271137.html, February 2023.

20   https://www.britishfibroidtrust.org.uk, February 2021.

21   'Medical Therapy', https://www.britishfibroidtrust.org.uk.

22   Patient Leaflet Mirena, https://www.medicines.org.uk, June
     2022.

23   Meyer, M., Sotres-Alvarez, D., 'Polycystic Ovary Syndrome
     Signs and Metabolic Syndrome in Premenopausal Hispanic/
     Latina Women: the HCHS/SOL Study', *Journal of Clinical
     Endocrinology and Metabolism*, 2020, 105(3), e447–56.

24   https://www.larabriden.com/cyclic-progesterone-therapy-
     for-pcos/, December 2022.

CHAPTER 8

1   Patient leaflet Microgynon 30, https://www.medicines.org.
     uk.

2   https://www.fsrh.org, February 2020.

3   https://www.stoptheclot.org.

4   Simon, J., 'What if the Women's Health Initiative had
     used transdermal estradiol and oral progesterone instead?'
     Menopause, 2014, 21(7),769–83.

5   Scarabin, P., 'Progestogens and venous thromboembolism in menopausal women: an updated oral versus transdermal estrogen meta-analysis', *Climacteric*, 2018,21(4), 341–5.

6   Patient Leaflet Yasmin, https://www.medicines.org.uk, August 2023.

7   McDaid, A., Logette, E., et al, 'Risk Prediction of Developing Venous Thrombosis in Combined Oral Contraceptive Users.' *PloS One*, 2017, 12, e0182041.

8   'Blood clot risks: comparing the AstraZeneca vaccine and the contraceptive pill', https://theconversation.com, April 2021.

9   McComish, H., *If Tits Could Talk*, (London, Cloc Book Print, 2023).

10   Holly McComish, youtube.com.

11   Hall, K. S., Trussell, J., 'Types of combined oral contraceptives used by US women', *Contraception*, 2012, 86(6), 659–65.

12   https://www.nih.gov/news-events/nih-research-matters/e-cigarettes-linked-blood-vessel-damage, November 2022.

13   https://www.frsh.org, April 2019.

14   Riccardi, M., Sammartino, A., 'Heart Failure: an update from the last years and a look at the near future', *ESC Heart Failure*, 2022, 9(6), 3761–3767.

15   https://researchbriefings.files.parliament.uk/documents/SN03336/SN03336.pdf, January 2023.

16   'Overweight & Obesity Statistics', USA, niddhk.nih.gov, 2021.

17   Fernandes, U., Guidi, G., et al, 'Breast cancer in young women: a rising threat: A 5-year follow-up comparative study', *Porto Biomedical Journal*, 2023, 8(3), e213.

18   https://www.fsrh.org, February 2020.

19   Fitzpatrick, D., Pirie, K., et al, 'Combined and progestagen-only hormonal contraceptives and breast cancer risk: A UK nested case–control study and meta-analysis' *Plos One*, 2023,1004188.

20   Leatham, X, 'Every type of the Pill or hormonal

contraception raises risk of breast cancer by up to a THIRD, major Oxford study reveals', dailymail.co.uk, March 2023.

21 Mørch L., Skovlund C., et al, 'Contemporary Hormonal Contraception and the Risk of Breast Cancer', *The New England Journal of Medicine*, 2017, 377(23), 2228–2239.

22 fsrh.org, March 2023.

23 Saul, H., Gursul, D., 'Risk of breast cancer with HRT depends on therapy type and duration', *BMJ,* 2022, 376, 0485.

24 Patient leaflet Dianette, https://www.medicines.org.uk, February 2023.

25 Shamseddin, M., De Martino, F., et al, 'Contraceptive progestins with androgenic properties stimulate breast epithelial cell proliferation', *EMBO Molecular Medicine*, 2021, 13, e14314.

26 Hultstrand, J. Gemzell-Danielsson, K., et al, 'Hormonal contraception and risk of breast cancer and breast cancer in situ among Swedish women 15–34 years of age: A nationwide register-based study', *The Lancet,* 2022, 21, 100470.

27 Fournier, A., Berrino, F., Clavel-Chapelon, F., 'Unequal risks for breast cancer associated with different hormone replacement therapies: results from the E3N cohort study', *Breast Cancer Research and Treatment*, 2008, 107(1), 103–11.

28 Britt, K., Short, R., 'The plight of nuns: hazards of nulliparity', *The Lancet*, 2012, 379(9834), 2322-3.

29 https://www.cancer.gov/about-cancer/causes-prevention/risk/hormones/oral-contraceptives-fact-sheet

30 Grabrick, D., Hartmann, L., Cerhan, J., et al, 'Risk of Breast Cancer With Oral Contraceptive Use in Women With a Family History of Breast Cancer', *JAMA,* 2000, 284(14), 1791–1798.

31 https://www.bcrf.org/blog/black-women-and-breast-cancer-why-disparities-persist-and-how-end-them/, Jan 2023.

32 Jemal, A., Robbins, A., 'Factors That Contributed to Black-White Disparities in Survival Among Nonelderly Women with Breast Cancer Between 2004 and 2013', *Journal of Clinical Oncology*, 2018, 36(1), 14–24.

33 Limb, M., 'Black women in England are at greater risk of late cancer diagnosis than white women', *BMJ,* 2023, 380, 211.

34 blackwomenrisinguk.org/about-us

35 Gowans-Eglinton, C., 'Why I stopped taking the pill and will never take it again', thetimes.co.uk, March 2023.

36 Duncan, C., 'Ultra-processed foods may be linked to increased risk of cancer', https://www.imperial.ac.uk, February 2023.

37 https://www.cancer.gov/about-cancer/causes-prevention/risk/hormones/reproductive-history-fact-sheet

38 https://www.cancer.gov/news-events/cancer-currents-blog/2020/breast-cancer-survival-exercise

39 Price, L., 'Dating After Cancer: Single, Bald, Female (30) Seeks...' https://www.huffingtonpost.co.uk, September 2013.

40 Price, L., *Single Bald Female*, (London, Macmillan, 2022).

41 Morimont, l., Haguet, H., 'Combined Oral Contraceptives and Venous Thromboembolism: Review and Perspective to Mitigate the Risk', *Frontiers in Endocrinology*, 2021, Sec. Reproduction, 12, 769187.

CHAPTER 9

1 https://www.naturalcycles.com/is-natural-cycles-right-for-me

2 Legal Terms, https://www.naturalcycles.com.

3 Venn, L., 'It's back: These are the influencers cashing in on the controversial Natural Cycles app', https://thetab.com, June 2021.

4 'Avoiding miscon(tra)ceptions', https://asa.org,uk, August 2018.

5 Fertility UK, https://www.fertilityuk.org

6 https://www.nhs.uk/conditions/contraception/natural-family-planning/

7 'FTC Finalizes Order with Flo Health, a Fertility-Tracking

App that Shared Sensitive Health Data with Facebook, Google, and Others', https://www.ftc.gov, June 2021.

8 Haridasani, A., Singer, N., 'Your App Knows You Got Your Period. Guess Who It Told?', https://www.nytimes.com/2021/01/28/us/period-apps-health-technology-women-privacy.html, January, 2021.

9 'No Body's Business But Mine: How Menstruation Apps Are Sharing Your Data', https://privacyinternational.org, 2018.

10 Shea, A., 'Scientific research at Clue: How tracking your cycle advances female health', https://helloclue.com/articles/about-clue/scientific-research-at-clue, August 2023.

CHAPTER 10

1 'FSRH CEU Clinical Statement: Contraceptive Choices and Sexual Health for Transgender and Non-Binary People', https://www.fsrh.org, October 2017.

2 Bailey, J., 'Sexual health needs of trans and non-binary people', *ResearchGate,* 2023, DOI:10.13140/RG.2.2.18778.93120.

3 The University of California at San Francisco, Transcare Guidelines, https://transcare.ucsf.edu.

4 Mancini, I., Alvisi, S., et al, 'Contraception across transgender' *International Journal of Impotence Research,* 2020 33(7), 710–719.

5 'Draft guideline on the "Care of Trans and Gender Diverse People within Obstetrics and Gynaecology" opens for consultation', rcog.org.uk, July 2022.

6 Nolan, I., Kuhner, C., Dy, G., 'Demographic and temporal trends in transgender identities and gender confirming surgery', *Translational Andrology and Urology,* 2019, 8(3):184–190.

7 https://www.thepinknews.com/2022/03/18/trans-sexual-health-clinics-lgbt/, March 2022.

8 Hibbert, M., Wolton, A., 'Exploring the low uptake of

sexual health services among trans people', *British Medical Journal* blog, November 2019.

9   'Cervical smears', https://www.dean.st.

10 'Masculinizing hormone therapy', https://www.mayoclinic. org, February 2023.

11 Panay, N., 'British Menopause Society Tools for Clinicians: Testosterone replacement in menopause', *Post Reproductive Health*, 2019, 25(1), 40–42.

12 Wierckx, K., Van Caenegem E., et al, 'Reproductive wish in transsexual men', *Human Reproduction*, 2012, 27(2), 483–7.

13 https://www.youtube.com/watch?v=7t76OxpZ4jo

14 'New STI data shows 24 per cent increase in rates in England', https://www.tht.org, June 2023.

15 https://www.thepinknews.com/2022/03/18/ trans-sexual-health-clinics-lgbt/

CHAPTER 11

1   'Medication Abortion Now Accounts for More Than Half of All US Abortions', https://www.guttmacher.org, February 2022.

2   https://www.gov.uk/government/statistics/abortion-statistics -for-england-and-wales-2021/abortion-statistics-england-and- wales-2021

3   Davies, M., 'Record number of abortions in Scotland', https://www.thetimes.co.uk, May 2023.

4   'What the data says about abortion in the U.S.', https://www. pewresearch.org, January 2023.

5   Schoenfeld Walker, A., McCann, A., 'Abortions Rose in Most States This Year, New Data Shows', https://www.nytimes. com, September 2023.

6   'The mental health impact of unplanned pregnancy and the right to abortion', https://www.bpas.org; Guttmacher.org; 'Nearly half of all pregnancies are unintended – a global crisis, says new UNFPA report', unfpa.org.

7   'Written Evidence from the British Pregnancy Advisory Service [WRH0036]', https://www.bpas.org.

8   Sanger-Katz, M., 'Who Gets Abortions in America?' https://
    www.nytimes.com, December 2021.

9   '9 in 10 UK adults now identify as pro-choice', https://www.
    msichoices.org, February 2020.

10 Ghorayashi, A., 'Puberty Starts Earlier Than It Used To. No
    One Knows Why', nytimes.com, May 2022.

11 Walker, N., 'My Abortion at 11 Wasn't a Choice. It Was My
    Life', https://www.nytimes.com, August 2022.

12 Rocca, C., Kimport, K., et al. 'Decision Rightness and
    Emotional Responses to Abortion in the United States: A
    Longitudinal Study', 2015, *Plos One,* 10(7), e0128832.

13 https://www.contraceptionchoices.org/contraceptive-method/
    condoms

14 Steinauer J., DePiñeres T., 'The importance of including
    abortion in undergraduate medical education', in: Landy U,
    Darney P.D., Steinauer, J. (Eds), *Advancing women's health
    through medical education: A systems approach in family planning and
    abortion,* (Cambridge University Press, 2021) 143–50.

15 https://www.gov.uk/government/statistics/abortion-statistics
    -for-england-and-wales-2021/abortion-statistics-england-and-
    wales-2021

16 https://www.rcog.org.uk/for-the-public/browse-our-patient-
    information/ectopic-pregnancy-patient-information-leaflet/

17 Oppenheim, M., 'I had an abortion – and my experience
    shows how broken the UK system truly is', https://www.
    independent.co.uk, March 2022.

18 'Six Months Post-Roe, 24 US States Have Banned Abortion
    or Are Likely to Do So: A Roundup', https://www.
    guttmacher.org, January 2023.

19 https://en.wikipedia.org/wiki/Manifesto_of_the_343

20 https://www.who.int/news-room/fact-sheets/detail/
    abortion

21 ibid.

22 McHugh, J., 'How 343 Women Made French History by
    Talking About Their Abortions', https://www.time.com,
    November 2018.

23 'Majority of Public Disapproves of Supreme Court's Decision To Overturn Roe v. Wade', https://www.pewresearch.org, August 2022.

24 Atwood, M., 'Enforced childbirth is slavery', https://www. theguardian.com, May 2022.

25 https://www.nytimes.com/interactive/2022/us/abortion-laws-roe-v-wade.html

26 Yang, M., 'Asian Americans do not have access to abortion information, survey finds', https://www.theguardian.com May 2023.

27 McCann, A., 'Inside the Online Market for Overseas Abortion Pills', nytimes.com April 2023.

28 Seitz, A., 'More women sue Texas, asking court to put emergency block on state's abortion law', apnews.com, May 2023.

29 https://www.contraceptionchoices.org/contraceptive-method/fertility-awareness

30 Haridasani, A., Singer, N., 'Your App Knows You Got Your Period. Guess Who It Told?', https://www.nytimes.com/2021/01/28/us/period-apps-health-technology-women-privacy.html, January 2021.

31 https://www.womensequality.org.uk/march_abortion_reform

32 Sinclair, L., 'Lily Allen: I wish people would stop posting examples of exceptional reasons for having abortions', https://www.stylist.co.uk/people/lily-allen-abortion-rights-comments/678091, 2021.

CHAPTER 12

1   Letter from Katherine McCormick to Margaret Sanger Nov 15, 1948 in *Ideas and Movements that Shaped America: From the Bill of Rights to 'Occupy Wall St'* Vol 1 edited by Michael Green, Scott L. Stabler (ABC-CLIO, Santa Barbara, California, 2015.) 147.

2   'Eugenics and Birth Control', pbs.org.

3   https://sanger.hosting.nyu.edu/documents/speech_morality_and_bc/

4   Stewart, N., 'Planned Parenthood in N.Y. Disavows
    Margaret Sanger Over Eugenics', https://www.nytimes.com,
    August 2020.

5   'Katharine Dexter McCormick: Fierce Feminist and Secret
    Smuggler', plannedparenthoodaction.org, August 2019.

6   Pendergrass, D., 'The Bitter Pill: Harvard and the Dark
    History of Birth Control', https://www.thecrimson.com,
    September 2017.

7   Garcia, C. R., Rock, J., Pincus, G., 'Effects of certain 19-
    Nor steroids on the normal human menstrual cycle', *Science*,
    1956, 124(3227), 891–3.

8   'Katharine Dexter McCormick', pbs.org.

9   ibid.

10 Pincus, G., 'Field Trials with Norethynodrel as an Oral
    Contraceptive', https://collections.countway.harvard.edu/
    onview/exhibits/show/conceiving-the-pill/item/6469

11 Vargas, T., 'Guinea pigs or pioneers? How Puerto Rican
    women were used to test the birth control pill', https://
    www.washingtonpost.com, May 2017.

12 Rock, J., Protocols, collections.countway.harvard.edu.

13 Sowemimo, A., *Divided: Racism, medicine and why we need to
    decolonise healthcare*, (London, Profile Books, 2023) 73.

14 ibid, 77.

15 'The Puerto Rico Pill Trials', https://www.pbs.org.

16 Vargas, T., 'Guinea pigs or pioneers? How Puerto Rican
    women were used to test the birth control pill', https://
    www.washingtonpost.com, May 2017.

17 Searle and Co, 'Enovid Medical Brochure', 1958, https://
    collections.countway.harvard.edu/onview/items/show/
    6470

18 Heggie, V., '54 years of the Pill (on the NHS), and how
    Birmingham women got it first', https://www.theguardian.
    com, December 2015.

19 ibid.

20 https://api.parliament.uk/historic-hansard/commons/1961/
    dec/04/birth-control-pills

21   http://93778645.weebly.com/letters-between-sanger-and-mccormick.html

22   Rock, J., 'It is not a foreign body once it gets into the feminine', https://collections.countway.harvard.edu/onview/items/show/6476

23   https://en.wikipedia.org/wiki/Humanae_vitae

24   Guillebaud, J., 'Reducing withdrawal bleeds', Correspondence, *The Lancet,* 2000, 355, 2169.

25   https://www.thecrimson.com/article/2017/9/28/the-bitter-pill/

26   Seaman, B., 'The Pill and I: 40 Years On, the Relationship Remains Wary', https://www.nytimes.com, May 2000.

27   Lyons, R., 'Panic and Pregnancies Linked To Senate Inquiry on Birth Pill', https://www.nytimes.com, February 1970.

28   https://en.wikipedia.org/wiki/Nelson_Pill_Hearings

29   'Senate Hearings on the Pill', pbs.org.

30   Wolfson, A., 'The Women's Movement Gave Me a Voice', interviewed by Judith Waxman, https://veteranfeministsofamerica.org/vfa-pioneer-histories-project-alice-wolfson/, June 2021.

31   Seaman, B., 'The Pill and I: 40 Years On, the Relationship Remains Wary', nytimes.com, June 2000.

CHAPTER 13

1   Shahvisi, A., 'Towards responsible ejaculations: the moral imperative for male contraceptive responsibility,' *Journal of Medical Ethics*, 2020, 46, 328–336.

2   Shahvisi, A., 'What can contraceptive justice teach us about coronavirus?', *Journal of Medical Ethics Forum*, March 2020.

3   https://www.plannedparenthood.org/learn/birth-control/withdrawal-pull-out-method/how-effective-is-withdrawal-method-pulling-out

4   Glasier, A., Anakwe, R., et al, 'Would women trust their partners to use a male pill?' *Human Reproduction*, 2000, 15(3), 646–9.

5   Reynolds-Wright, J., Cameron, N., Anderson, R.,

'Will Men Use Novel Male Contraceptive Methods and Will Women Trust Them?' *The Journal of Sex Research*, 2021, 58 (7), 838–849.

6 Nguyen, B., Jacobsohn, T., 'Men's willingness to use novel male contraception is linked to gender-equitable attitudes: Results from an exploratory online survey', *Contraception*, 2023, 123, 110001.

7 'Permanent Contraception and Restrictive Abortion Laws: Trends in Vasectomies After the Overturn of Roe v. Wade', https://www.komodohealth.com, April 2023.

8 'Trends in U.S. Adolescent Sexual Behavior and Contraceptive Use, 2006-2019', https://www.guttmacher.org, April 2021.

9 https://www.hanxofficial.com, November 2021.

10 https://www.tht.org.uk/news/new-sti-data-shows-24-increase-rates-england, June 2023.

11 'STI Increase: Syphilis cases spike 74 per cent in four years', https://www.healthline.com, April 2023.

12 https://graziadaily.co.uk/life/in-the-news/stealthing-conviction-rape/, April 2019.

13 'What comes in 66 sizes and vegan latex? The new generation of condoms', https://www.theguardian.com, October 2017.

14 'A non-hormonal pill could soon expand men's birth control options', https://www.acs.org, March 2022.

CHAPTER 14

1 Audre Lorde, *The Cancer Journals*, (San Francisco, Aunt Lute Books,1977), 7.

2 'Unlocking opportunities in women's healthcare', https://www.mckinsey.com, February 2022.

3 https://popcouncil.org/media/celanese-announces-agreement-with-the-population-council-for-sustained-release-dual-api-therapeutic/, 2023.

4 Schimpf, U., Caldas-Silveira, E., 'Topical reinforcement of the cervical mucus barrier to sperm', *Science Translational Medicine*, 2022, 14(673).

5 Fletcher, J., Yee, H., Ong, B., Roden, R. C., 'Centering disability visibility in reproductive health care: Dismantling barriers to achieve reproductive equity', *Womens Health (London)*, 2023, 19:17455057231197166.

6 Fruzzetti, F., Cagnacci, A., 'Venous thrombosis and hormonal contraception: what's new with estradiol-based hormonal contraceptives?', *Open Access Journal of Contraception*, 2018, 9, 75–79.

7 Robertson, E., Kulkarni, J., et al, 'Pilot Data on the Feasibility And Clinical Outcomes of a Nomegestrol Acetate Oral Contraceptive Pill in Women With Premenstrual Dysphoric Disorder' *Frontiers in Endocrinology*, 2021, 12, 70448.8

8 Mu, E., Kulkarni, J., 'Hormonal contraception and mood disorders', *Australian Prescriber*, 2022, 45(3), 75–79.

9 Tiranini, L., Cucinella, L., et al, 'Is now the time to reconsider risks, benefits, and limitations of estrogen preparations as a treatment for menstrually related migraine?', *Expert Review of Neurotherapeutics*, 2023, 23(4), 377–388.

10 Eisenlohr-Moul, T., Bowers, S., Prinstein, M., et al, 'Effects of acute estradiol and progesterone on perimenstrual exacerbation of suicidal ideation and related symptoms: a crossover randomized controlled trial', *Translational Psychiatry*, 2023, 12, 528.

11 Gates, M., *The Moment of Lift: How Empowering Women Changes the World*, (New York, Flatiron Books, 2019).

INDEX